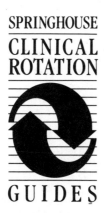

SPRINGHOUSE
CLINICAL
ROTATION

GUIDES

MW00906458

# NEUROLOGIC-NEUROSURGICAL NURSING

Mary Jane Evans, RN, BSN, CCRN

Springhouse Corporation
Springhouse, Pennsylvania

# Staff For This Volume

## CLINICAL STAFF

**Clinical Director**
Barbara F. McVan, RN

**Clinical Editors**
Joanne Patzek DaCunha, RN, BS;
Joan E. Mason, RN, EdM; Diane
Schweisguth, RN, BSN,
CCRN, CEN

## PUBLICATION STAFF

**Executive Director, Editorial**
Stanley Loeb

**Executive Director, Creative Services**
Jean Robinson

**Design**
John Hubbard (art director),
Stephanie Peters (associate art
director), Jacalyn Bove Facciolo

**Editing**
Susan L. Taddei (senior acquisitions
editor), David Prout, Bernadette M.
Glenn (acquisitions assistant)

**Copy Editing**
Katherine Tsioulcas (manager), Nick
Anastasio, Keith de Pinho, Elizabeth
B. Kiselev, Diane Labus, Doris
Weinstock, Debra Young

**Art Production**
Robert Perry (manager), Loretta
Caruso, Anna Brindisi, Donald
Knauss, Robert Wieder

**Typography**
David Kosten (manager), Diane
Paluba (assistant manager), Nancy
Wirs, Brenda Mayer, Joyce Rossi
Biletz, Robin Rantz

**Manufacturing**
Deborah Meiris (manager), T.A.
Landis

**Project Coordination**
Aline S. Miller (supervisor), Laurie J.
Sander

Library of Congress Cataloging-in-Publication Data
Evans, Mary Jane
    Neurologic-neurosurgical nursing. Mary Jane
    Evans.
        p. cm. — (Clinical rotation guides)
    Bibliography: p.
    Includes index.
    ISBN 0-87434-172-8
    1. Neurological nursing.  I. Title.  II. Series.
    [DNLM:  1. Nervous System Diseases —
    nursing.   2. Neurosurgery—nursing.
    WY 160 E923]
RC350.5.E9 1988
610.73'68—dc19
DNLM/DLC
for Library of Congress                          88-20026
                                                        CIP

To Mary and Albert Romeo

# Special Acknowledgment

The author wishes to thank Florida Hospital, Orlando, Florida, owned and operated by the Adventist Health System, for the services and support that made this series possible.

### Series Consulting Editor
**Mary Jane Evans, RN, BSN, CCRN**
    Independent Consultant for Nursing Education

### Clinical Consultant
**Corey H. Evans, MD**
    Associate Director
    Family Practice Residency
    Florida Hospital
    Orlando, Fla.

# Table of Contents

# Advisory Board

## Neurologic-Neurosurgical Nursing

**Marie Scott Brown, RN, PhD**
Professor of Nursing
Family Nursing Department
School of Nursing
University of Oregon Health Sciences Center
Portland, Ore.

**Lillian S. Brunner, RN, MSN, ScD, LittD, FAAN**
Nurse-Author
Brunner Associates, Inc.
Berwyn, Pa.

**Charmaine J. Cummings, RN, MSN**
Clinical Nurse Educator
Neurology, Eye, and Aging Nursing Research Service
National Institutes of Health
Bethesda, Md.

**Joanne V. Hickey, RN, BSN, MSN, MA, PhD**
Professor of Nursing and Independent Consultant in
    Neuroscience Nursing
Community College of Rhode Island
Warwick, R.I.

**Celestine B. Mason, RN, BSN, MA**
Associate Professor
School of Nursing
Pacific Lutheran University
Tacoma, Wash.

**William L. Shopp, RN, BSN, CNRN**
Head Nurse
Neurosurgical Intensive Care
Cleveland Clinic Hospital
Cleveland, Ohio

**Carol E. Smith, RN, PhD**
Professor
School of Nursing
University of Kansas
Kansas City, Kan.

**Connie A. Walleck, RN, MS, CNRN**
Associate Director of Nursing
Maryland Institute for Emergency Medical Services
Baltimore, Md.

# Preface

This book, designed as a supplementary aid, will assist the student in planning and implementing nursing care of the neurologic-neurosurgical patient in the clinical setting. It in no way substitutes for an in-depth study of neurologic patient care but provides quick information useful to nursing students on neurology-neurosurgery clinical rotations. Within this book, the student will find clinical instruction on:

1. performing a neurologic admission assessment and providing ongoing neurologic observation and evaluation

2. understanding the essential concepts of terms frequently used in neurology and neurosurgery

3. assisting with or performing neurologic-neurosurgical procedures and diagnostic tests

4. preparing nursing diagnoses and interventions for neurologic diseases and disorders using the nursing process

5. understanding and using specialized neurologic-neurosurgical equipment

6. managing preoperative and postoperative care for the neurosurgical patient

7. caring for patients with head and spinal injuries

8. managing neurologic-neurosurgical emergencies

9. understanding neurologic drugs, their dosage, action, and nursing implications.

# 1 Essentials of Neurologic Assessment

Medical management of the neurologic patient concentrates on diagnosing and treating neurologic deficits. Nursing management, by comparison, focuses on detecting changes in the neurologic status of these patients and preventing further loss of function from neurologic deficits.

Because you must evaluate a hospitalized neurologic patient frequently, you won't have time to conduct a complex, lengthy examination each time. Instead, you'll monitor his condition for changes by:
• establishing a baseline of neurologic function at admission
• conducting routine neurologic checks (abbreviated but frequent neurologic assessments usually documented in checklist form).

We'll discuss neurologic checks in more detail beginning on page 13, but first, let's discuss how to establish baseline assessment findings.

## ☐ Baseline Admission Assessment

A neurologic admission assessment establishes a baseline of neurologic function for both conscious and unconscious patients. You'll gauge subsequent improvement or deterioration by comparing changes in the patient's status with admission assessment findings. The admission evaluation includes a neurologic nursing history and physical assessment.

### Neurologic Nursing History

Neurologic patients may have memory loss or other impaired thought processes. Before obtaining the admission history, establish the patient's reliability by interviewing the family or someone familiar with his previous behavior. Record the family's perception of the patient's mental status.

As part of your routine nursing history, be sure to include the following items, which are important in assessing the neurologic patient and in helping plan patient care:
• past or present problems with motor function (including paralysis), sensation, memory, thought processes, speech function, or intellectual function as well as fainting spells, dizziness, headache, cancer, seizures, or head injury
• social history (education, employment, alcohol consumption, and family history of neurologic disorders)
• sleep disturbances (wandering behavior, insomnia, daytime sleepiness, or sleep apnea)

• personality changes (confusion, lethargy, depression, mood swings, or belligerent behavior)
• bowel or bladder incontinence
• medications (tranquilizers, sedatives, or anticonvulsants)
• allergies.

## Physical Assessment

Although less extensive than a complete medical neurologic examination, your initial physical assessment is more detailed than a neurologic check. Besides a routine review of all body systems, your initial physical should include the following items of particular significance to neurologic patients.

### Vital signs

**Pulse,** if abnormal and combined with other neurologic signs and symptoms, may indicate serious neurologic problems. For example, a slow pulse and a widening pulse pressure (difference between systolic and diastolic blood pressure) suggest increasing intracranial pressure (ICP).

**Respirations** should be recorded, noting the rate, depth, rhythm, and breathing pattern. Changes in any of these may indicate dysfunction of hemispheric structures or the brain stem. Five pathologic respiratory patterns may help identify areas of brain injury (see page 3):
• Cheyne-Stokes breathing
• central neurogenic hyperventilation
• apneustic breathing
• cluster breathing
• ataxic breathing.

**Blood pressure** is regulated by the brain stem. If ICP increases, the brain stem may become compressed or even herniate through the foramen magnum, causing severe neurologic dysfunction or death. Widening pulse pressure with a slowing pulse rate may warn of impending brain stem damage.

**Temperature elevation,** with its accompanying rise in metabolic rate, decreases the amount of oxygen available to the brain. Neurologic patients require nursing interventions aimed at keeping their temperature within normal limits. Although fever usually indicates infection, hypothalamic dysfunction is another possible cause.

### Mental status

Establishing the patient's mental status on admission is a critical part of the neurologic exam. One of the first signs of cerebral dysfunction is a change in mental status, which can be assessed by the following indicators.

**Orientation** involves the patient's awareness of person, place, and time. Ask the patient who he is (person), where he is (place), and what day it is (time). If he answers all three questions correctly, write "oriented × 3" on the record. Keep in mind that any patient can easily become disoriented to time in a hospital; therefore, consider disorientation to time less significant than disorientation to person or place.

**Level of consciousness** is determined by the patient's awareness and responsiveness to his environment. Consciousness ranges from alert

## ABNORMAL BREATHING PATTERNS ASSOCIATED WITH BRAIN INJURY

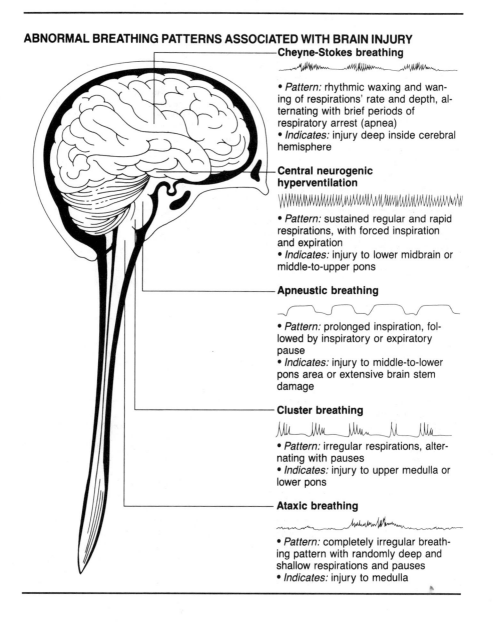

**Cheyne-Stokes breathing**

• *Pattern:* rhythmic waxing and waning of respirations' rate and depth, alternating with brief periods of respiratory arrest (apnea)
• *Indicates:* injury deep inside cerebral hemisphere

**Central neurogenic hyperventilation**

• *Pattern:* sustained regular and rapid respirations, with forced inspiration and expiration
• *Indicates:* injury to lower midbrain or middle-to-upper pons

**Apneustic breathing**

• *Pattern:* prolonged inspiration, followed by inspiratory or expiratory pause
• *Indicates:* injury to middle-to-lower pons area or extensive brain stem damage

**Cluster breathing**

• *Pattern:* irregular respirations, alternating with pauses
• *Indicates:* injury to upper medulla or lower pons

**Ataxic breathing**

• *Pattern:* completely irregular breathing pattern with randomly deep and shallow respirations and pauses
• *Indicates:* injury to medulla

## MEDICAL AND COLLABORATIVE MANAGEMENT OF INCREASED INTRACRANIAL PRESSURE

| Treatment | Purpose | Nursing considerations |
|---|---|---|
| Restriction of fluid | Reduces cerebral edema by reducing total body water | • Monitor fluids and electrolytes (including osmolarity) closely. Dehydration below 325 Osm may have little therapeutic value.<br>• Maintain fluid restrictions according to the doctor's orders. (He'll probably restrict an adult patient to 1,200 or 1,500 ml/day.)<br>• Document the patient's fluid intake and output accurately. Remember to include all I.V. medications in your calculations. |
| Administration of steroids I.V.; for example, dexamethasone (Decadron) | Reduces cerebral edema by lowering sodium and water concentration in the brain | • Give steroid with antacids orally and cimetidine (Tagamet) orally or I.V., as ordered, to prevent peptic ulcers.<br>• Watch for signs and symptoms of gastrointestinal bleeding, such as dark-colored stools, low blood pressure, dizziness, nausea, and vomiting large amounts of bright red blood. |
| Hyperventilation with hand-held resuscitator | Helps blow off $CO_2$ which causes constriction of blood vessels and reduction of cerebral blood flow | • Monitor arterial blood gas measurement. Notify the doctor if $CO_2$ continues to rise. He may want to increase the rate of ventilations. |
| Administration of osmotic diuretics, for example, mannitol (Osmitrol) by I.V. drip or bolus | Reduces cerebral edema by shifting fluid from intracellular to intravascular space for elimination | • Monitor fluids and electrolytes (including osmolarity) closely. Treatment may cause rapid dehydration.<br>• Watch for a rebound rise in intracranial pressure (ICP) from treatment.<br>• Avoid storing mannitol at low temperatures, as it may crystallize. |
| Administration of barbiturates to induce coma; for example, phenobarbital (Luminal) | Decreases cerebral metabolic rate; decreases cerebral blood flow | • Monitor vital signs regularly, especially respirations.<br>• Give barbiturates, as ordered. Remember, when performing neurologic checks on your patient, you'll have difficulty assessing his mental status when he's receiving barbiturates. |
| Withdrawal of cerebrospinal fluid (CSF) by performing a lumbar or cisternal puncture, or using a ventricular catheter | Reduces CSF volume | • If the doctor performs a lumbar or cisternal puncture, perform neurologic checks frequently after the procedure. Remember, a sudden drop in ICP may allow brain herniation.<br>• If the doctor uses a ventricular catheter, prevent sepsis by changing the tubing and drainage bag using strict aseptic technique. |
| Surgical removal of skull bone flap | Allows for expansion of cranial contents | • Keep site clean and dry to prevent infection.<br>• Maintain strict aseptic technique when redressing the site. |

to comatose, but the following terms are intended only as guidelines for classifying a patient's response to his environment. When assessing and recording level of consciousness, explicitly record the stimulus used and the patient's response to it.

*Alertness.* An alert patient responds appropriately to external stimuli. Alertness is the "normal" state of an awake individual to which other levels of consciousness are compared. Alert patients may be oriented or disoriented.

*Lethargy.* A lethargic (obtunded) patient appears indifferent and has slow, quiet, and sometimes incomplete responses. He drifts back to sleep soon after he's awakened. Like alert patients, lethargic patients can be oriented or disoriented. Motor responses are slowed and delayed when the patient withdraws from noxious stimuli or reacts to verbal or tactile stimulation.

## UNDERSTANDING INCREASED INTRACRANIAL PRESSURE

Intracranial pressure (ICP) is the pressure that the intracranial contents exert against the cranial vault. Intracranial contents normally include brain tissue, blood, and cerebrospinal fluid (CSF), and may include hematomas, abscesses, tumors, and fluid surrounding injured tissue (edema). Because the skull is an inflexible vault, if the intracranial contents expand, ICP rises, compressing the brain and causing tissue damage and dysfunction. The skull has only one opening at its base, the foramen magnum. With increased ICP, the brain stem may herniate (push through) this opening. Because the brain stem controls such vital functions as respiration and blood pressure, this complication usually proves fatal.

*To assess for increased ICP*
Conduct neurologic checks every 30 to 60 minutes, as ordered, or more frequently if changes are detected. Watch for these signs and symptoms of increased ICP:
• a change in the patient's level of consciousness, including loss of consciousness
• a pupil that dilates or fails to react to light (see page 15)
• pronounced changes in vital signs, especially widening pulse pressure
• sudden onset of signs and symptoms indicating severe neurologic deficit, such as

hemiparesis, hemiplegia, facial paralysis, slurred speech, and abnormal posturing (in a comatose patient).

*To prevent or manage increased ICP*
• Prevent hypercapnia (PaCO$_2$ >45 mm Hg) and hypoxia (PaO$_2$ <60 mmHg).
• Limit the patient's fluid intake, as ordered.
• Position him to avoid neck flexion and head rotation.
• Advise him not to perform Valsalva's maneuver.
• Don't permit long, uninterrupted periods of activity; allow him to rest between nursing procedures.
• Elevate the head of the bed 30 degrees (unless contraindicated).
• Control fever and keep the patient quiet.

*Medical interventions*
The doctor may initiate ventricular, subarachnoid, or epidural monitoring to detect the earliest signs of increased ICP (see *Three Types of ICP Monitoring,* page 94). To relieve increased ICP in an emergency, he may remove CSF from the ventricles through a small twist drill hole in the skull, a procedure called ventriculostomy. Keep a ventriculostomy tray at hand, in case of emergency. For a chart of other medical interventions, see *Medical and Collaborative Management of Increased Intracranial Pressure.*

*Stupor.* A stuporous patient responds only to vigorous and continuous noxious stimuli, such as knuckles rubbed forcefully against the sternum. He can't talk but makes purposeful movements to stop the painful stimuli.

*Coma.* A comatose patient has completely lost consciousness and cannot be aroused. Reflexes may be present (moderate coma) or absent (deep coma).

## Cranial nerve function

Most of the cranial nerves originate in the brain stem, which contains structures essential for maintaining life and consciousness. Specifically, the brain stem controls respiratory rate, depth, and pattern and such cardiovascular activities as blood vessel constriction. The reticular activating system, which maintains consciousness, is also located in the brain stem.

Evaluating brain stem function is critical because its malfunction endangers consciousness and may prove fatal. To assess brain stem function at the bedside, evaluate the cranial nerves listed below (which are both named and designated by Roman numerals).

You needn't assess all cranial nerves. You can rapidly obtain a reliable indication of brain stem function from this examination. (For a complete cranial nerve examination, see pages 7 and 8.)

**Optic (II).** Ask the patient if he's having any vision problems, or test his vision.

**Optic (II) and oculomotor (III).** Check pupillary size, shape, and reaction to light. Pupils should be round and should constrict equally and bilaterally when exposed to light. To conduct the examination, shine a light to the side of the patient's head, and holding each eyelid open, pass it directly in front of each pupil. Constriction of that pupil is called *direct response.* Then, holding both eyelids open with one hand, pass the light in front of one pupil while observing the other. Constrictive response in the pupil away from the light is called *consensual response.* Both responses are normal. Record the specific size and shape of each pupil, approximating its size using a pupillary chart (see page 9), and record whether or not they react equally.

**Oculomotor (III), trochlear (IV), and abducens (VI).** Check external eye movements by having the patient's eyes follow your finger above, below, and to the right and left while keeping his head stationary. Move your finger toward the midline of his face and observe for convergence (movement of eyes toward the midline). In the unconscious patient you can test for the oculocephalic reflex, as shown on page 9.

*(continued on page 9)*

## CRANIAL NERVE ASSESSMENT

To perform a thorough neurologic examination, assess the 12 paired cranial nerves, classified as motor nerves, sensory nerves, or both motor and sensory nerves.

| | Cranial nerve | Assessment |
|---|---|---|
| 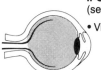 | **I-Olfactory**<br>(sensory)<br><br>• Smell | Have the patient close his eyes. Occlude one nostril with your finger, and ask him to identify nonirritating odors, such as coffee, tea, cloves, soap, chewing gum, and peppermint. Repeat the test on the other nostril. |
|  | **II-Optic**<br>(sensory)<br><br>• Vision | Assess visual acuity with a Snellen chart or newspaper. Or ask the patient to count how many fingers you're holding up. Check visual fields by confrontation. Have the patient sit directly in front of you and stare at your nose. Slowly move your finger from the periphery toward the center until the patient says he can see it. Check color vision by asking the patient to name the color of several nearby objects. |
| 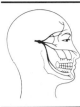 | **III-Oculomotor**<br>(motor)<br><br>• Pupillary constriction<br>• Upper eyelid elevation<br>• Most eye movement<br><br>**IV-Trochlear**<br>(motor)<br><br>• Downward and inward eye movement<br><br>**VI-Abducens**<br>(motor)<br><br>• Lateral eye movements | The motor functions of these nerves overlap, so test them together. First, inspect the eyelids for ptosis. Then assess ocular movements by moving your finger to each quadrant of the visual field with the patient's eyes fixed on your finger, and note any eye deviation. Test accommodation and direct and consensual light reflexes. |
|  | **V-Trigeminal**<br>(both)<br><br>• Sensation to the corneas, nasal and oral mucosa, and facial skin<br>• Mastication | To test motor function, ask the patient to close his jaws tightly. Then try to separate his clenched jaw. Also test the corneal reflex by lightly touching the patient's cornea with a cotton wisp. To check this nerve's sensory function, ask the patient to close his eyes. Then lightly touch his forehead, cheeks, and chin. Can he feel the touch equally on both sides? |
| | **VII-Facial**<br>(both)<br><br>• Facial muscles<br>• Taste perception (on the tongue's anterior two thirds) | Have the patient show his teeth, attempt to close his eyes against resistance, and puff out his cheeks. Then dab sugar, salt, or vinegar on the front of his tongue. Have the patient identify these substances by their taste. |

*(continued)*

## CRANIAL NERVE ASSESSMENT *(continued)*

| Cranial nerve | Assessment |
|---|---|
| **VIII-Acoustic**<br>(sensory)<br><br>• Hearing (cochlear)<br>• Equilibrium (vestibular)<br>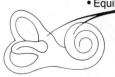 | Rub a few strands of hair between your fingers next to the patient's ear. Then have him identify which ear you selected. Also check his ability to hear a watch ticking or a whisper. Observe the patient's balance. Does he sway when walking or standing? Perform a Romberg test, if indicated. |
| **IX-Glossopharyngeal**<br>(both)<br><br>• Swallowing and phonation<br>• Sensation to the pharyngeal, soft palate, and tonsillar mucosa<br>• Taste perception (on the tongue's posterior third)<br>• Salivation<br>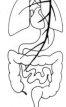<br>**X-Vagus**<br>(both)<br><br>• Swallowing and phonation<br>• Sensation to the exterior ear's posterior wall and behind the ear<br>• Sensation to the thoracic and abdominal viscera | First, have the patient identify tastes at the back of his tongue. Then inspect the soft palate. Observe for symmetrical elevation when the patient says *aah.* Touch the soft palate's mucous membrane with a swab to elicit the palatal reflex. Touch the posterior pharyngeal wall with a tongue depressor to elicit the gag reflex. |
| **XI-Spinal accessory**<br>(motor)<br><br>• Uvula and soft palate movement<br>• Sternocleidomastoid muscle<br>• Upper portion of trapezius muscle (governs shoulder movement and neck rotation)<br>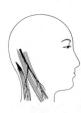 | Palpate and inspect the sternocleidomastoid muscle as the patient pushes his chin against your hand. Palpate and inspect the trapezius muscle as the patient shrugs his shoulders against your resistance. Also have the patient stretch out his hands toward you. |
| **XII-Hypoglossal**<br>(motor)<br><br>• Tongue movements involved in swallowing and speech<br>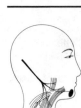 | Observe the tongue for asymmetry, atrophy, deviation to one side, and fasciculations. Ask the patient to push his tongue against a tongue depressor. Then have him move his tongue rapidly in and out and from side to side. |

**Facial (VII).** Have the patient smile, and check for facial asymmetry. Assess facial sensation.

**Trigeminal (V).** Ask the patient to make chewing movements with his jaw. Check mouth and nose sensation.

**Vagus (X).** Insert a tongue depressor in the patient's mouth and touch the posterior pharynx. Observe for the gag reflex. Look for symmetrical elevation of the soft palate when the patient says "aah."

## DOCUMENTING PUPIL SIZE

Use this chart as a guide to documenting your patient's pupil size. Remember, normal pupil size is 2 to 6 mm, with 3.5 mm the average.

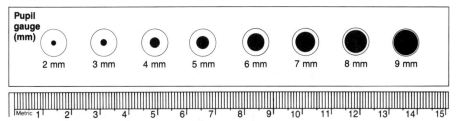

## DOLL'S EYE REFLEX
(OCULOCEPHALIC REFLEX)

How can you quickly assess brain stem function in an unconscious patient? Test his oculocephalic reflex, which is sometimes called doll's eye reflex. To test for this reflex, hold the patient's eyelids open. Then, quickly—but gently—turn his head to the right. If everything's OK, his eyes will appear to move conjugately toward the center of his body (left of his eye sockets). But if his eyes remain stationary in the center or to the right of his eye sockets, his doll's eye reflex is absent, indicating a deteriorating consciousness level. Notify the doctor.

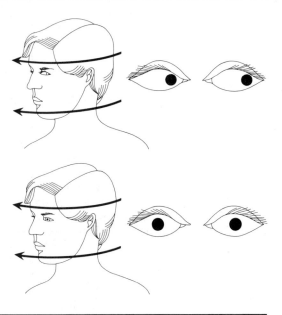

## ICE WATER CALORICS (OCULOVESTIBULAR REFLEX)

This procedure, an indicator of brain stem function, tests the oculov-estibular reflex by checking the condition of nerve fibers between the brain and the semicircular canals (cranial nerve VIII). The patient's external ear canal is irrigated with cool water via a 50-ml syringe. Normally, the patient's eyes move slowly toward the irrigated ear and rapidly back to mid-position. Abnormal responses include:
• absence of movement, suggesting brain stem failure
• eyes remaining longer in the direction of the irrigated ear, also sug-gesting brain stem malfunction
• normal slow phase of movement toward irrigated ear without rapid return, suggesting bilateral cerebral hemisphere dysfunction (sluggish return movement).

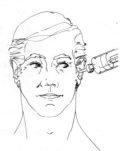

## Motor function

For a motor response to occur, nerve pathways from the brain to end organs and muscles must be intact. The upper motor neu-rons originate in the cerebral cortex and end at various levels in the spinal cord, where they synapse directly or via spinal inter-neurons with lower motor neurons. Upper motor neurons are re-sponsible for initiating voluntary movement. Lower motor neurons originate at various levels in the spinal cord and termi-nate on the muscle. They transmit upper motor neuron impulses or can be part of a motor reflex. Evaluate motor nerve function by assessing muscle movement and strength.

Start by having the patient simultaneously squeeze both of your hands with his hands. Evaluate the strength of the grip in both hands; document his grip as equal or unequal, strong or weak. Evaluate subtle extremity weakness and problems with proprioception by checking for *arm drift:* Have the patient stand with his hands ex-tended outward (perpendicular to the body) and with his eyes closed. An affected arm slowly drifts down. In the comatose patient, strength and grip cannot be tested voluntarily.

Ask the patient to move all his extremities. Record the presence or absence of movement or any unilateral or bilateral weakness. Deter-mine whether movement is spontaneous or in response to command. Is spontaneous movement against gravity? Can the patient move an extremity against mild, moderate, or forceful resistance? An entry might read, "Patient moves all E's in response to command, against gravity, and against moderate resistance."

Testing the patient's motor reflexes reveals the condition of sensory and motor pathways to and from muscle tendons and muscles to the spinal cord and brain. When a clinician taps on a muscle tendon (such as the one beneath the patella) with a re-flex hammer, he is observing for an immediate, controlled jerk of the extremity in response to his action. A normal knee-jerk reflex indicates that the neural pathways to and from the spinal cord to the muscle and tendon are intact.

## TESTING DEEP TENDON REFLEXES

You'll need a percussion hammer to test your patient's tendon reflexes. Test each reflex bilaterally as follows:

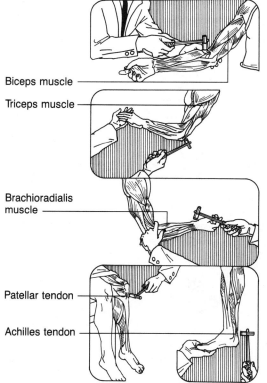

Biceps muscle

Triceps muscle

Brachioradialis muscle

Patellar tendon

Achilles tendon

**Biceps reflex**
Rest the patient's elbow in your hand. Position your thumb over his biceps tendon. Then percuss your thumbnail and watch for forearm flexion.

**Triceps reflex**
Flex the patient's arm slightly, using your hand to steady his arm. Percuss the tendon above the back of his elbow. Watch for elbow extension.

**Brachioradialis reflex**
Ask the patient to rest his hand on his thigh with the hand positioned as shown. Percuss the radius and watch for forearm flexion.

**Patellar reflex**
Have the patient sit on a table with his legs dangling freely (or have him cross his legs). Percuss the tendon right below his patella. Watch for leg extension at the knee.

**Achilles reflex**
Support the patient's foot in your hand. Rotate his foot and leg outward and percuss the Achilles tendon. Watch his ankle for plantar flexion.

Reflex tests such as this one are important in localizing damage or injury to nervous tissue. If any reflex is absent, it usually indicates a lower motor neuron problem, that is, a problem originating in the motor nerve of the reflex arc.

Hyperreflexia (an abnormally intense response to a stimulus) indicates a lesion of the upper motor neurons, which carry impulses from the brain to the lower motor neurons. Hyperreflexia suggests a lack of cortical control over the reflex. The illustration on page 13 shows how reflexes are elicited and graded.

### Sensory function

Ask an alert patient if he has experienced any unusual sensations, such as numbness or tingling, anywhere in his body. Test sensation perception using sharp (pinprick) and dull (finger) stimulation over the area in question. Always test with the patient's eyes closed.

## THE REFLEX ARC

Stretching a muscle tendon by tapping it with a reflex hammer excites the sensory neurons in the muscle and tendon, creating an impulse. In the muscle stretch reflex, the sensory neurons synapse directly with *lower motor neurons* and the impulse results in an immediate motor response, like the quick knee jerk from testing the patellar reflex. When a lower motor neuron is damaged, we would expect to see sluggishness or absence of the reflex response.

The reflex arc is modulated by neurons from the brain. These *upper motor neurons* extend from the cerebral cortex to the motor nerve, exerting a dampening effect on the reflex. For example, hyperreflexia would likely be an upper motor neuron problem, because lack of cortical control over the reflex has caused a hyperactive motor response to the stimulus.

## BABINSKI'S REFLEX

When you test your patient for Babinski's (or plantar) reflex, you are looking for voluntary motor dysfunction that originates in the corticospinal tract or motor area of the cerebrum.

Stroke the lateral aspect of the sole of your patient's foot (left). The normal response is flexion of the toes (center). If the Babinski's reflex is present, the great toe will dorsiflex and the other toes will fan apart (right). This response indicates an upper motor neuron lesion.

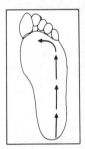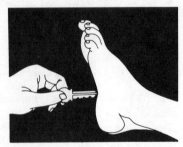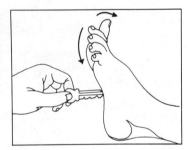

When assessing the patient in stupor or coma, apply forceful pressure to the nail beds, or rub the sternum vigorously with your knuckles and observe his response, if any.

### Coordination and balance

Balance and coordination are indicators of cerebellar function. To evaluate coordination, hold your index finger about 15 inches from the patient's face. Instruct him to touch your fingertip with his index finger and then touch the tip of his nose. He should do this repeatedly in rapid succession. Assess the movement's accuracy and smoothness. To evaluate balance, have the patient walk heel-to-toe across the room and assess his stability.

## TESTING AND GRADING REFLEXES

Testing and grading muscle stretch reflexes helps determine whether the neurologic problem is originating in upper or lower motor neurons. It also reveals the condition of the reflex pathway at the level where the patient is being tested. This examination procedure is referred to as eliciting DTRs (deep tendon reflexes), and responses are graded according to the following scale:

*Muscle stretch reflex grades*
  0   absent
  1+  present but diminished
  2+  normal
  3+  increased but not
necessarily pathologic

  4+  hyperactive; clonus may also be present

*Superficial reflex grades*
  0   absent
  ∓   equivocal or barely present
  +   normally active

Record the patient's reflex scores by drawing a stick figure and entering the scores at the proper location. The figure shown here indicates normal muscle stretch reflex activity, as well as normal superficial reflex activity over the abdominal area.

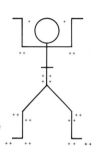

---

# ☐ Ongoing Assessment and Neurologic Checks

As mentioned earlier, besides taking the baseline admission assessment, the nurse must evaluate the neurologic patient routinely for changes in neurologic status. The doctor determines the minimum number of neurologic checks to be performed per hour or shift.

Neurologic check findings are sometimes recorded on a clinical flow sheet for convenience and easy access (see page 14). Also document vital signs and any other routine neurologic assessment findings the doctor requests. In a routine neurologic check, you'll assess:

**Orientation** to person, place, and time and level of consciousness (ranging from alertness to coma). Note the patient's speech: Is it clear? rambling? slurred? Can he follow commands?

**Response to noxious stimuli** in the comatose patient. Note his movements: Are they purposeful (tries to push your hand away when you elicit the pain response) or nonpurposeful (restless flailing movements)?

**Pupils** (size, shape, equality, and speed of response to light). Observe the patient's eye movement: Do you see nystagmus (rapid and repeated involuntary movement of the eyes)? Do his eyes deviate from the midline?

**Handgrip strength** and extremity movements. Are grips equal? Weak? Can the patient move his extremities against gravity? Against resistance (your hands pushing against them)?

## SAMPLE FLOW CHART FOR NEUROCHECK

Use the following chart to perform a neurocheck on your patient.

| **Will awaken to** | | | | | | | | |
|---|---|---|---|---|---|---|---|---|
| Name | | | | | | | | |
| Shaking | | | | | | | | |
| Light pain | | | | | | | | |
| Moderate pain | | | | | | | | |
| Deep pain | | | | | | | | |
| **Consciousness** | | | | | | | | |
| Oriented | | | | | | | | |
| Disoriented | | | | | | | | |
| Restless | | | | | | | | |
| Combative | | | | | | | | |
| **Speech** | | | | | | | | |
| Clear | | | | | | | | |
| Rambling | | | | | | | | |
| Garbled | | | | | | | | |
| None | | | | | | | | |
| **Pupils** | | | | | | | | |
| Size on right | | | | | | | | |
| Size on left | | | | | | | | |
| Reaction on right | | | | | | | | |
| Reaction on left | | | | | | | | |
| **Motor reaction to pain** | | | | | | | | |
| Appropriate | | | | | | | | |
| Inappropriate | | | | | | | | |
| None | | | | | | | | |
| **Ability to move** | | | | | | | | |
| Arms—Normal power | | | | | | | | |
| Mild weakness | | | | | | | | |
| Severe weakness | | | | | | | | |
| Spastic flexion | | | | | | | | |
| Extension | | | | | | | | |
| No response | | | | | | | | |
| Legs—Normal power | | | | | | | | |
| Mild weakness | | | | | | | | |
| Severe weakness | | | | | | | | |
| Spastic flexion | | | | | | | | |
| Extension | | | | | | | | |
| No response | | | | | | | | |

## Assessing the Comatose Patient

When assessing a comatose patient, evaluation of pupils and motor function deserves special attention.

Continually assess a comatose patient for signs of increased ICP. Observe his pupils for signs of impending brain stem herniation. Single pupil dilation, bilateral fixed dilation, or loss of reactivity to light may indicate herniation. Notify the doctor immediately if you see these signs.

The response of a comatose patient to noxious stimuli (such as rubbing your knuckles forcefully on his sternum or squeezing

### UNDERSTANDING PUPILLARY CHANGES

Use this chart as a guide to what your patient's pupillary changes may signify.

| Pupil description | Possible causes |
|---|---|
| Dilated, unilateral, fixed, no reaction to light   | • Uncal herniation with oculomotor nerve damage<br>• Brain stem compression due to an expanding mass lesion or an aneurysm<br>• Increased intracranial pressure<br>• Tentorial herniation<br>• Head trauma with subsequent subdural or epidural hematoma |
| Dilated, bilateral, fixed, no reaction to light   | • Severe midbrain damage<br>• Cardiopulmonary arrest (hypoxia)<br>• Anticholinergic poisoning |
| Midsized, bilateral, fixed, no reaction to light   | • Midbrain involvement due to edema, hemorrhage, infarctions, lacerations, contusions |
| Pinpoint, usually bilateral, no reaction to light   | • Lesion of pons, usually after hemorrhage, leading to blocked sympathetic impulses<br>• Opiates (morphine)—pupils may be reactive |
| Small, unilateral, no reaction to light   | • Disruption of sympathetic nerve supply to head due to spinal cord lesion above T1 |

his Achilles tendon) may indicate the nature of the lesion. Therefore, you must report explicitly and accurately all motor responses to stimuli as well as the type of stimulus used to elicit
the response. Watch for the following abnormal responses:

**Paratonic rigidity,** an early indicator of cerebral dysfunction in
which motor responses range from resistance to passive motion
of the extremities to intense rigidity of the entire body.

**Mass response,** a motor response to a stimulus that involves the
comatose patient's entire body. (See *Recognizing Abnormal Postures* below for examples.) Mass responses can be of three types:
*Decorticate posturing,* in which the patient flexes his arms,
wrists, and fingers in response to a stimulus and exhibits leg extension and plantar flexion.
*Decerebrate posturing,* in which the patient extends his head
and neck and adducts, extends, and pronates his arms. Also expect plantar flexion and extension of the lower legs. Decerebrate
posturing may occur in response to stimuli, spontaneously, or
continuously.
*Opisthotonos,* an arching of the neck and spine, most commonly
seen in seizures and severe meningeal irritation.

## RECOGNIZING ABNORMAL POSTURES

A patient exhibiting any of the three abnormal postures described here may have severe neurologic damage. If your patient assumes any of these postures, alert the doctor immediately.

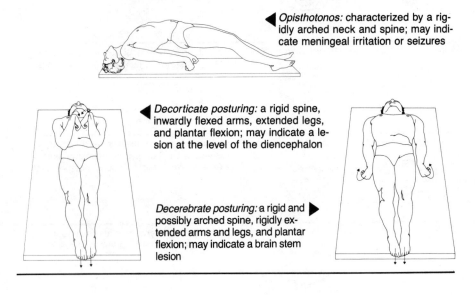

◀ *Opisthotonos:* characterized by a rigidly arched neck and spine; may indicate meningeal irritation or seizures

◀ *Decorticate posturing:* a rigid spine,
inwardly flexed arms, extended legs,
and plantar flexion; may indicate a lesion at the level of the diencephalon

*Decerebrate posturing:* a rigid and ▶
possibly arched spine, rigidly extended arms and legs, and plantar
flexion; may indicate a brain stem
lesion

# 2 Diagnostic Tests and Nursing Interventions

The following diagnostic tests and nursing interventions are arranged in alphabetical order.

## ☐ Angiography, Cerebral

### Purpose
To locate cerebrovascular abnormalities.

### Procedure
Patient is injected with contrast medium via the carotid, femoral, or brachial artery in order to obtain a series of cerebrovascular X-rays.

### Patient preparation
• Explain that the test, which lasts about 2 hours, examines the brain's blood circulation. The patient will be injected with a contrast medium that makes the blood vessels visible on X-rays.
• Do not permit food or fluids 8 to 10 hours before the test.
• Make sure the patient has signed a consent form.
• Remove jewelry and other radiopaque objects.
• Ask the patient about allergies to iodine and iodine-containing substances such as shellfish. Report allergies to doctor.
• Administer premedication 30 to 45 minutes before the procedure.

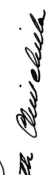

### Post-test care
• If the carotid artery was used as the injection site:
 —observe for dysphagia or respiratory distress, which may indicate internal bleeding and tracheal compression.
 —observe for disorientation, weakness, sensory changes, or transient neurologic deficits, which may indicate a thrombus, an occlusion, or spasm of the carotid artery.
 —check the injection site for hematoma.
• If the femoral artery was used as the injection site:
 —keep the affected leg straight and pressure dressing over puncture site for 12 hours.
 —take the dorsalis pedis and popliteal pulses every 2 to 4 hours.
 —note any temperature or color changes in the leg.
 —check the injection site for hematoma.
• If the brachial artery was used as the injection site:
 —immobilize the arm and keep pressure dressing in place over puncture site for 12 hours.
 —take the radial pulse every 2 to 4 hours.
 —don't take blood pressures on the affected arm.

—note any temperature or color changes in the arm.
—check the injection site for hematoma.
• Regardless of which approach was used:
—check vital signs and perform neurologic checks at least every hour for the first 4 hours, then on a routine basis.
—provide an ice bag for swelling at the injection site.

# ☐ Brain Scan, Radioisotope

## Purpose
To diagnose masses, vascular lesions, and ischemic or infarcted areas in the brain.

## Procedure
A radionuclide bolus is injected into the antecubital vein. Rapid X-rays are taken as the isotope passes through the brain. The scanner produces images that may reveal tissue or blood flow abnormalities.

## Patient preparation
• Explain that the test helps to detect abnormalities in the brain and its blood vessels. This essentially painless and harmless procedure lasts about 1½ hours.
• Inform the patient that no food or fluid restrictions are necessary.
• Remove jewelry and other radiopaque objects.

## Post-test care
Observe the injection site for possible hematoma, and treat with cold pack, if necessary.

# ☐ Brain Stem Auditory Evoked Response

## Purpose
To test the eighth cranial nerve, considered one of the last portions of the brain stem to remain intact in cases of severe brain stem deterioration.

## Procedure
An electrode is placed deep in the ear canal. Surface scalp electrodes record electrically evoked responses. These responses appear as electrical sequelae on computer-averaged electroencephalograms.

## Patient preparation
This test requires no patient preparation or cooperation because it is usually administered to comatose or obtunded patients.

## Post-test care
No intervention is required.

# ☐ Computed Tomography (CT) Scan

## Purpose
To diagnose intracranial lesions or to determine the extent of intracranial injury. To monitor effects of chemotherapy or radiotherapy.

## Procedure
The patient lies immobile on the table with his head stationary inside the scanner. X-rays are taken at 1-degree intervals in a 180-degree arc. Contrast medium is injected, if ordered, and another series of X-rays are taken.

## Patient preparation
• Explain that the test is a type of computerized X-ray that detects brain abnormalities and lasts about 15 to 30 minutes.
• No food or fluid restrictions are necessary unless contrast medium is used. If an "enhanced" study (one that uses contrast medium) is ordered, restrict food and fluids for 4 hours.
• Make sure that the patient has signed a consent form for contrast studies.
• Ask the patient about allergies to iodine or iodine-containing substances, such as shellfish.

## Post-test care
• CT scans have no known complications if contrast agents are not used.
• The patient may experience nausea and vomiting or headache from contrast agents. If asymptomatic, the patient may resume his previous diet.

# ☐ Digital Subtraction Angiography

## Purpose
To visualize cerebral blood flow and detect vascular abnormalities, such as aneurysms, tumors, and hematomas.

## Procedure
This type of intravenous angiography combines X-ray methods and a computerized subtraction technique so that vessels may be visualized without interference from bone or other soft tissue. The interfering structures are "subtracted" (removed) from the image by a computer.

## Patient preparation
• Explain that a contrast medium will be injected into a vein and X-rays taken in order to detect abnormalities in the head or neck.
• Inform the patient that the procedure lasts about 1 hour.
• Ask the patient about allergies to iodine or other contrast media and report allergies to the doctor.

### Post-test care
• The risk of arterial bleeding (as in regular angiography) is eliminated because the dye is injected into a vein.
• Vital signs should be checked and neurologic checks performed every 30 minutes during the first hour, then routinely.

## ☐ Echoencephalography

### Purpose
To detect a major shift in midline cerebral structures indicating a possible lesion.

### Procedure
A transducer is placed on the temporal area and emits an ultrasonic beam that is reflected off midline brain structures, indicating the distance from the transducer to cerebral structures.

### Patient preparation
• Explain that the test determines the position of certain structures within the brain, that no pain is involved, and that the test lasts about 1 hour.
• Inform the patient that no food or fluid restrictions are necessary.

### Post-test care
This noninvasive procedure has no complications, but it has largely been replaced by CT scans.

## ☐ Electroencephalography (EEG)

### Purpose
To evaluate the brain's electrical activity in various neurologic disorders—for example, providing a differential diagnosis of epilepsy.

### Procedure
Electrodes (usually flat, but sometimes needle electrodes) are placed on the scalp. The EEG records electrical brain activity while the patient is lying down or sitting in a recliner.

### Patient preparation
• Explain that electrodes will be placed on the scalp to detect brain activity. Although the patient must remain relaxed and still, EEG is a painless procedure that lasts about 30 minutes.
• Check with the doctor about discontinuing anticonvulsants and sedatives before the test.
• Inform the patient that no food or fluid restrictions are necessary.

### Post-test care
Check with the doctor about reinstating discontinued medications.

## ☐ Electromyography

### Purpose

To differentiate muscle disease from nervous disorders and to diagnose neuromuscular disorders, such as myasthenia gravis.

### Procedure

Needle electrodes are placed in the muscles to be tested in order to record their electrical signals during rest and contraction.

### Patient preparation

• Explain that the test measures electrical activity of muscles and that needles will be inserted into various muscles and their electrical response recorded. The procedure is not usually painful, although it may cause some discomfort. Inform the patient that the test lasts about 1 hour.
• Inform the patient that no food or fluid restrictions are usually necessary.
• Check with the doctor about withholding coffee, other sources of caffeine, and cigarettes.

### Post-test care

• Provide analgesics and warm compresses if the patient complains of residual pain.
• Resume withheld substances, if approved by the doctor.

## ☐ Lumbar Puncture

### Purpose

To measure cerebrospinal fluid (CSF) pressure and to obtain CSF specimens for laboratory analysis.

---

### POSITIONING THE PATIENT FOR LUMBAR PUNCTURE

Have the patient lie on his side at the edge of the bed, with his chin tucked to his chest and his knees drawn up to his abdomen. Make sure the patient's spine is curved and his back is at the edge of the bed, as shown here. This position widens the spaces between the vertebrae, facilitating insertion of the needle.

To help the patient maintain this position, place one of your hands behind his neck and the other hand behind his knees, and pull gently. Hold the patient firmly in this position throughout the procedure to prevent accidental needle displacement.

Fourth lumbar vertebra
Third lumbar vertebra
Subarachnoid space

## CEREBROSPINAL FLUID FINDINGS

| Test | Normal | Abnormal | Implications |
|------|--------|----------|--------------|
| Pressure | 50 to 180 mm H$_2$O | Increase | Increased intracranial pressure from hemorrhage, tumor, or edema caused by trauma |
| | | Decrease | Spinal subarachnoid obstruction above puncture site |
| Appearance | Clear, colorless | Cloudy | Infection (elevated white blood cell [WBC] count and protein, or many micro-organisms) |
| | | Xanthochromic or bloody | Subarachnoid, intracerebral, or intraventricular hemorrhage; spinal cord obstruction; traumatic tap (usually noted only in initial specimen) |
| | | Brown, orange, or yellow | Elevated protein, red blood cell (RBC) breakdown (blood present for at least 3 days) |
| Protein | 15 to 45 mg/100 ml | Marked increase | Tumors, trauma, hemorrhage, diabetes mellitus, polyneuritis, blood in cerebrospinal fluid (CSF) |
| | | Marked decrease | Rapid CSF production |
| Gamma globulin | 3% to 12% of total protein | Increase | Demyelinating disease (such as multiple sclerosis), neurosyphilis, Guillain-Barré syndrome |
| Glucose | 50 to 80 mg/100 ml (⅔ of blood glucose) | Increase | Systemic hyperglycemia |
| | | Decrease | Systemic hypoglycemia, bacterial or fungal infection, meningitis, mumps, post-subarachnoid hemorrhage |
| Cell count | 0 to 5 WBCs | Increase | Active disease: meningitis, acute infection, onset of chronic illness, tumor, abscess, infarction, demyelinating disease (such as multiple sclerosis) |
| | No RBCs | RBCs | Hemorrhage or traumatic tap |
| VDRL and other serologic tests | Nonreactive | Positive | Neurosyphilis |
| Chloride | 118 to 130 mEq/liter | Decrease | Infected meninges (as in tuberculosis or meningitis) |
| Gram stain | No organisms | Gram-positive or gram-negative organisms | Bacterial meningitis |

## Procedure

The procedure is usually performed in the patient's bed. Position the patient on his side with his back at the edge of the bed, as shown below. Help him maintain this knee-chest position throughout the procedure by placing one arm around his knees and the other around his neck. The area (usually between the third and fourth lumbar vertebrae) is prepared, draped, and anesthetized using 1% or 2% lidocaine. A spinal needle is inserted and the stylet removed. A manometer with stopcock is attached to the needle and the pressure is measured. (See *Cerebrospinal Fluid Findings*.) The stopcock is opened and specimens are collected. Another pressure measurement is taken before the needle is removed. An adhesive bandage is placed over the puncture site. Alternate methods that are rarely used for obtaining CSF include ventricular puncture and cisternal puncture.

### Patient preparation

• Explain that a needle will be inserted into the lower back to measure fluid pressure in the spine and to withdraw CSF for laboratory analysis.
• No food or fluid restrictions are necessary.
• Make sure the patient has signed a consent form.
• Prepare a lumbar puncture tray, including gloves, lidocaine, povidone-iodine solution, and adhesive bandages.

### Post-test care

• Keep the patient flat in bed for 8 hours after the procedure unless otherwise ordered.
• Perform neurologic checks at least every hour for the first 4 hours. (If CSF pressure is elevated, perform them more frequently.)
• Encourage the patient to drink fluids, if not contraindicated.
• Observe the puncture site for signs of bleeding, redness, swelling, and drainage every 4 hours for 24 hours.
• Provide analgesics for headache.

# ☐ Magnetic Resonance Imaging (MRI)

## Purpose

To image brain anatomy in order to diagnose tumors, infarcts, vascular malformations, and other abnormalities.

## Procedure

The patient is placed under a strong magnetic field and pulsed with a radio frequency. The body's soft tissues release their own radio frequencies that are used to develop an image.

## Patient preparation

• Explain that the test is similar to an X-ray and can detect brain abnormalities, although it uses no radiation. MRI is painless and lasts approximately 15 to 30 minutes.

• No food or fluid restrictions are necessary.
• MRI is contraindicated for patients with pacemakers, metallic clips for cerebral aneurysms, or prosthetic heart valves.

### Post-test care
This noninvasive procedure has no known complications.

## ☐ Myelography

### Purpose
To diagnose lesions within the spinal cord (such as tumors) and herniated intervertebral disks.

### Procedure
A lumbar puncture is performed, and CSF is withdrawn for analysis. The table is tilted with the patient lying prone. Contrast medium is injected into the subarachnoid space and allowed to displace CSF, following the course of gravity. The contrast medium's flow is studied for obstruction, using fluoroscopy. X-rays are taken for the patient record.

### Patient preparation
• Explain that the test, which lasts about 1½ hours, locates obstructions in the spinal cord.
• Inform the patient that no food or fluids should be consumed 8 hours before the test; however, if the test is late in the day, clear liquids may be consumed.
• Make sure the patient has signed a consent form.
• Administer the premedication as ordered, 30 to 45 minutes before the procedure.

### Post-test care
• Check orders for positioning (varies with contrast medium used).
• Check vital signs and perform neurologic checks every 30 minutes for the first 2 hours, then on a routine basis.
• Encourage fluids, if not contraindicated.
• Have the patient void within 8 hours after the procedure.
• Observe for meningeal signs (see page 63).
• Administer analgesics for headache as ordered.

# 3 Neurologic Disorders and the Nursing Process

When caring for the neurologic patient, the nurse should be aware of general signs and symptoms associated with nervous tissue dysfunction. Regardless of the specific neurologic disease or disorder the patient is experiencing, the signs and symptoms are related to the extent of nervous tissue damage.

Disease or injury may cause nervous tissue destruction, damage, or irritation. When nervous tissue is *destroyed,* permanent paralysis and loss of sensation result. When nervous tissue is *damaged,* total paralysis and loss of sensation may result, but partial or complete recoveries frequently occur. When nervous tissue is *irritated,* as when a misaligned vertebra compresses a spinal nerve, numbness and tingling of the associated nerve endings result. If brain tissue becomes irritated, as in infection, seizures may occur. Regardless of the patient's diagnosis, paralysis, loss of sensation, numbness, tingling, and seizure activity as well as changes in the level of consciousness and orientation are the hallmarks of nervous tissue damage or dysfunction. As your experience with neurologic patients increases, you will find that no matter what the damage, the nervous system can produce only a limited number of abnormal signs and symptoms.

The following disorders are arranged in alphabetical order.

## ☐ Alzheimer's Disease

Alzheimer's disease is the most common cause of dementia. It involves neuronal degeneration throughout the cerebral cortex. Associated dysfunction and neurologic deficits manifest as memory and behavioral changes. Motor and sensory impairment may also occur.

### Assessment

#### Frequently encountered subjective data
• memory changes
• fatigue
• complaints of weakness and impaired motor skills

#### Frequently encountered objective data
• insidious decline in capabilities and thought processes
• suspiciousness and fearfulness related to imaginary people and situations
• misperception of the environment
• misidentification of objects and people
• complaints of misplaced or stolen objects

• overdependence on significant others
• inability to use correct words, often with substitution of meaningless words
• conversations that drift into nonsensical phrases
• gradual loss of reading and writing ability
• emotional lability that may include inappropriate laughing and crying, mood swings, sudden angry outbursts, and sleep disturbances
• hoarding of inanimate objects
• aimless wandering
• disorientation to time and place (orientation to person usually stays intact until late in the disease)
• recent memory impairment (remote memory typically remains intact)
• inability to do simple calculations or repeat the names of three or more objects
• impaired motor skills
• loss of autonomic function control (bowel and bladder incontinence)

## Nursing Diagnosis

Alteration in Thought Processes: Disorientation related to inability to evaluate reality.
*Desired outcome:* Patient's periods of transient disorientation will be minimized.

### Interventions and rationales

1. Use soft tones and a slow, calm manner when speaking.
*Rationale:* Patient tends to misperceive stimuli and may feel threatened by loud, aggressive vocal tones.
2. Give simple directions, using easily understandable words and sentences.
*Rationale:* Impairment of the brain's communication centers reduces the patient's ability to decipher complex messages.
3. Allow the patient to keep personal belongings at the bedside.
*Rationale:* This prevents feelings of isolation and deprivation and enhances the patient's sense of self. It also aids in recall and reality orientation.
4. Call the patient by name whenever possible.
*Rationale:* This establishes and maintains a sense of identity and individual recognition.

## Nursing Diagnosis

Alteration in Thought Processes: Disruptive Behavior related to misperception of reality.
*Desired outcome:* Patient's agitated or combative behavior will be eliminated or minimized.

### Interventions and rationales

1. Maintain a quiet environment.
*Rationale:* Crowds, clutter, and noise may result in a distorted input that can confuse and irritate the patient.
2. Respond to the patient's questions with meaningful statements, giving the patient positive feedback whenever possible.
*Rationale:* Simple, concrete replies directly related to the patient's questions decrease frustration and anger.
3. Avoid criticism and arguments that lead to confrontations.
*Rationale:* The patient easily feels threatened. Any provocation may trigger anger or combative behavior.
4. Permit the patient to hoard inanimate objects.
*Rationale:* Hoarding seems to counterbalance mental and physical losses and gives the patient a sense of security. Removing these items is very disturbing to the patient and often results in disruptive behavior.

## Nursing Diagnosis

Alteration in Thought Processes: Memory Deficit related to inability to recall recent events secondary to cerebral cortical degeneration.
*Desired outcome:* Patient's recall of recent events will improve with reality orientation.

### Interventions and rationales

1. Provide orientation aids, such as clocks, pictures of family, and calendars.
*Rationale:* These items reinforce reality and help fill memory gaps.
2. Allow the patient to relate stories, for example, about his children and grandchildren.
*Rationale:* This helps the patient adjust to his changed environment. Past persons, places, and events in the patient's life can be used to relate to present reality and help in orienting the patient.

## Nursing Diagnosis

Diversional Activity Deficit related to decreased attention span.
*Desired outcome:* The patient will participate in activities compatible with his capabilities.

### Interventions and rationales

1. Provide an opportunity for the patient to engage in activities involving movement, such as short walks and outings.
*Rationale:* This preserves mobility and reduces the risk of bone and muscle atrophy. In addition, it provides mild sensory stimulation that frequently has a positive effect on orientation and cognitive function (attention span).

2. Ensure that activities fall within the patient's capabilities.
*Rationale:* The patient may feel threatened and frustrated by activities that lead to failure. Participating in activities (including diversional and self-care activities) daily reinforces feelings of usefulness and worth.

## Nursing Diagnosis
Alteration in Thought Processes: Ineffective Rest-Activity Pattern related to disorientation.
*Desired outcome:* The patient's wandering will be reduced or managed, and a rest-activity pattern will be established.

### Interventions and rationales
1. Schedule frequent rest periods, if possible; avoid activities that require concentration late in the day.
*Rationale:* Confusion increases with fatigue.
2. Avoid using restraints.
*Rationale:* Restraints commonly increase agitation and impede rest.

## Nursing Diagnosis
Potential for Physical Injury related to impaired judgment.
*Desired outcome:* Patient safety is maintained. Patient will sustain no injury as a result of his mental condition.

### Interventions and rationales
1. Minimize potential environmental hazards, for example, by forbidding unsupervised smoking; cigarettes and matches should not be permitted in the patient's room.
*Rationale:* Impaired judgment can lead to accidental injury; a disoriented patient cannot evaluate unforeseen consequences, such as an accidental fire caused by a misplaced cigarette.
2. Keep medications, poisons, and hazardous substances away from the patient.
*Rationale:* A patient who tampers with objects may place them in his mouth.
3. Teach the patient's family how to avoid potential hazards at home.
*Rationale:* An unsupervised patient cannot provide for his basic safety needs.
4. Stay alert for nonverbal clues.
*Rationale:* The patient may have expressive aphasia and sensory loss and, frequently, may express pain by doubling over or indicate thirst by sucking his fist or panting. If these clues are not detected by health care personnel, physical injury may result.

## Nursing Diagnosis

Self-Care Deficit (specify bathing/hygiene, dressing/grooming, toileting, or feeding) related to disorientation, confusion, and/or memory loss.

*Desired outcome:* The patient will participate in self-care activities to the extent of his capabilities.

### Interventions and rationales

1. Encourage patient independence.

*Rationale:* This promotes self-esteem and eases frustration over functional deficits.

2. Allow the patient ample time to perform tasks.

*Rationale:* The patient has decreased motor skills and frequently suffers mental and physical fatigue.

3. If you attempt to help the patient with activities of daily living and he becomes combative, postpone the activity.

*Rationale:* The patient's anger is quickly forgotten because of short-term memory impairment, so you can probably resume the activity in a few moments.

## Nursing Diagnosis

Altered Nutrition: Less than Body Requirements: Decreased Intake related to impaired judgment, motor deficits, and/or disorientation.

*Desired outcome:* The patient's nutritional balance will be maintained.

### Interventions and rationales

1. Allow the patient to feed himself to the extent to which he is capable.

*Rationale:* This decreases possible conflicts during meals; patients refuse to eat when they're irritable or angry.

2. Allow the patient ample time to eat. Cut his food and provide finger foods when possible.

*Rationale:* Impaired motor function requires more time to complete tasks. Finger foods allow more independence at mealtime and less potential conflict.

3. Provide assistance with menu selection.

*Rationale:* The patient becomes easily overwhelmed by choices, and his confusion usually makes him unaware of basic nutritional needs.

## Nursing Diagnosis

Altered Bowel Elimination: Constipation or Diarrhea related to loss of neuromuscular functioning and/or disorientation.

*Desired outcome:* Elimination problems will be controlled.

### Interventions and rationales

1. Take the patient to the bathroom at least every 2 hours.
*Rationale:* A regular schedule helps prevent accidents in cases of loose stools and encourages regularity in cases of constipation.
2. Make sure the patient knows where the bathroom is located. Color code the door or post a sign, if necessary.
*Rationale:* This enhances the patient's orientation.
3. Encourage sufficient fluid intake (2 liters/day) and a high-fiber diet in cases of constipation.
*Rationale:* This promotes evacuation and proper stool consistency.
4. Have patient use disposable underpants if he is ambulatory.
*Rationale:* These underpants will prevent potentially embarrassing accidents and save nursing time.

## Nursing Diagnosis

Ineffective Family Coping related to patient's disruptive behavior.
*Desired outcome:* The family copes effectively with the patient's long-term incapacitation.

### Interventions and rationales

1. Include the patient's family in planning home care.
*Rationale:* Knowing the family's life-style, resources, and special needs is essential in planning the patient's care. A cooperative plan established by the nurse reduces the family's burden.
2. Provide comfort and support to the patient's family.
*Rationale:* Caring for the patient involves much self-sacrifice by the family. Acquaint them with homemaker services or a local chapter of the Alzheimer's Disease and Related Disorders Association, and counsel them about day care and respite care services.

## Medical Diagnosis

**Laboratory tests,** such as complete blood count (CBC), VDRL test, vitamin $B_{12}$ and electrolyte levels, and thyroid studies, can detect potentially reversible nutritional, endocrine, and infectious disorders.

**Electroencephalography (EEG)** may reveal a generalized slowing of the brain waves, which supports the diagnosis.

**Hearing and vision testing** rules out altered sensory perception as the etiology.

**Computed tomography (CT) scan** may show characteristic ventricular widening and cortical atrophy, eliminating other causes of mental deterioration, such as a tumor or an abscess.

### Medical treatment

Medical treatment is supportive. No recognized cure or treatment exists for Alzheimer's disease.

| FAMILY COPING | ALZHEIMER'S DISEASE |

*Whenever possible, actively involve the patient and family or signifi-cant other in discussing:*

• the progressive decline of mental and physical abilities associ-ated with the disease and the need to establish a plan for care during the later stages, such as adult day care or home health care
• diagnostic tests—the purpose, procedure, and how to obtain the results
• the importance of a daily routine of care and physical activity
• dietary problems, such as dysphagia, malnutrition, and dehydra-tion
• techniques for establishing bladder and bowel regimens
• methods of managing confusion and home safety measures
• medications—actions, side effects, and administration
• the importance of time away from the patient for the primary care-giver
• local sources of additional help, such as home health care and support groups.

## ☐ Amyotrophic Lateral Sclerosis

Amyotrophic lateral sclerosis (ALS) involves degeneration of up-per motor neurons in the cortex and brain stem and lower mo-tor neurons in the spinal cord. This degeneration results in progressive muscular atrophy. ALS (also known as Lou Gehrig's disease) usually occurs between the ages of 40 and 70; patients have a 3- to 10-year life expectancy after onset.

### Assessment

#### Frequently encountered subjective data
• generalized weakness, especially in the small hand muscles
• difficulty speaking
• difficulty chewing
• difficulty breathing
• choking or fear of choking
• depression
• muscle weakness

#### Frequently encountered objective data
• spontaneous contractions of individual muscle fibers (fasciculations)
• loss of muscle mass
• muscle weakness
• impaired speech
• impaired breathing
• choking
• depression

## Nursing Diagnosis

Ineffective Airway Clearance related to dysphagia.
*Desired outcome:* No signs or symptoms of partial or complete airway obstruction (coughing, inability to talk, or choking) will occur. If they do, they will be managed promptly.

### Interventions and rationales

1. Feed the patient slowly.
*Rationale:* Muscle atrophy makes it more difficult to swallow food and coordinate breathing.
2. Discourage the patient from talking while eating.
*Rationale:* The patient must concentrate on coordinating his swallows with breathing to avoid airway obstruction.
3. Keep suction equipment at the bedside, and suction as needed.
*Rationale:* Suctioning helps remove accumulated secretions.
4. Teach the patient how to suction himself.
*Rationale:* Having a suction machine readily accessible at home reduces the patient's fear of choking. Using the suction machine in the hospital will familiarize the patient with the procedure.
5. Give the patient soft, solid foods and position him upright during meals.
*Rationale:* Soft, solid foods are easier to swallow, and sitting upright helps prevent possible aspiration. If aspiration occurs, causing complete occlusion, the Heimlich maneuver is employed, as with any complete airway obstruction. An unsuccessful Heimlich manuever is followed by the obstructed airway sequence of basic life support.

## Nursing Diagnosis

Impaired Skin Integrity related to immobility.
*Desired outcome:* No signs or symptoms of skin breakdown (redness, tissue thinness, petechiae, blistering, or necrosis) will occur.

### Interventions and rationales

1. Change the patient's position every 2 hours if he cannot do so himself.
*Rationale:* This prevents pressure sores by relieving or reducing pressure on bony prominences.
2. Maintain dry skin.
*Rationale:* Moisture increases the risk of bacterial growth and tissue breakdown.
3. Massage around bony prominences.
*Rationale:* This increases circulation to these areas and prevents ischemic breakdown.
4. Pad bony prominences wherever possible.
*Rationale:* This helps distribute pressure evenly and protects the skin.

5. Place the patient on a turning frame, flotation mattress, sheepskin pad, silicone pad, or split-foam mattress. Place a pillow between his knees.
*Rationale:* These measures distribute body weight more evenly and prevent pressure over bony prominences.
6. Inspect the patient's skin for signs of breakdown once every 8 hours.
*Rationale:* Early detection of skin breakdown improves the chance for successful treatment.

## Nursing Diagnosis
Self-Care Deficit (specify bathing/hygiene, dressing/grooming, toileting, or feeding) related to muscle atrophy.
*Desired outcome:* The patient will perform self-care confidently within the limits of his ability.

### Interventions and rationales
1. Assess the patient's capacity to perform activities of daily living. Assist him with bathing, personal hygiene, and transfer from wheelchair to bed only as needed.
*Rationale:* The patient must learn new techniques to compensate for loss of muscle strength.
2. Help the patient obtain assistive equipment, such as a walker or a wheelchair, to use in the hospital and later at home.
*Rationale:* ALS is a progressive, degenerative illness, and the patient will need to have necessary equipment at home and be familiar with its use.
3. Arrange for a visiting nurse to evaluate the patient's status, provide support, and continue to teach the patient and family about the illness.
*Rationale:* Continuing evaluation, support, and teaching are necessary to fulfill the patient's changing needs.
4. Provide emotional support and prepare the patient and family for his eventual death.
*Rationale:* ALS usually causes death 3 to 10 years after onset.
5. If the patient's condition allows, implement a rehabilitation program with the family that helps maintain the patient's independence as long as possible.
*Rationale:* This improves the patient's self-concept and diminishes feelings of frustration and depression.

## Nursing Diagnosis
Dysfunctional Grieving: Depression related to loss of body function.
*Desired outcome:* No signs or symptoms of depression (loss of appetite, difficulty sleeping, poor self-esteem, frequent crying spells) will occur, or if they do, they will be recognized and treated promptly. The patient will verbalize an understanding of the signs and symptoms of clinical depression.

## Interventions and rationales

1. Provide a supportive atmosphere.
*Rationale:* Lack of emotional support contributes to depression.
2. Listen attentively to the patient's feelings and concerns; do not dispute or negate them.
*Rationale:* Verbalizing situational factors is often helpful for the patient.
3. Help the patient reach a realistic assessment of his situation.
*Rationale:* The patient must gradually accept that ALS is a progressively degenerative and eventually fatal disease.
4. Encourage meaningful activity that offers the patient an opportunity for achievement compatible with his level of function.
*Rationale:* Achievement enhances the patient's self-esteem.
5. Encourage adequate rest.
*Rationale:* ALS causes weakness and fatigue, which reduce the patient's coping ability.
6. Refer the patient to a psychiatric nurse specialist, if needed.
*Rationale:* This is a chronic degenerative disease with a poor prognosis requiring extensive follow-up care and long-term evaluation.

## Medical Diagnosis

**Electromyography and muscle biopsy** differentiate nerve from muscle disease.

**Lumbar puncture** determines the protein content of cerebrospinal fluid (CSF), which increases in one third of ALS patients.

**CT scan** rules out spinal cord neoplasm and lesions compressing the spinal cord.

### Medical treatment

No effective medical treatment is currently available for ALS.

---

**FAMILY COPING**  **AMYOTROPHIC LATERAL SCLEROSIS**

*Whenever possible, actively involve the patient and family or significant other in discussing:*

• the progressive nerve and muscle degeneration associated with the disease and the need to establish a plan for care during the later stages, such as a nursing care facility or home health care
• the signs and symptoms of clinical depression and when to seek professional help
• diagnostic tests—the purpose, procedure, and how to obtain results
• the importance of exercise to prevent muscle atrophy in unaffected muscles
• dietary adjustments, such as using semisoft foods for dysphagia
• suctioning technique for removing secretions and emergency procedures for choking

• feeding techniques if the patient is discharged with a gastros-
tomy or nasogastric tube
• alternate communication techniques if the patient's vocal cords
are affected
• the importance of family time away from the patient if they are the
primary caregivers.

## ☐ Aneurysm, Cerebral

Cerebral aneurysm is a localized dilatation, or ballooning, of a
cerebral artery, caused by a weakness in the vessel wall. It is
seen most commonly at the arterial junctions in the circle of Willis, the circular anastomosis, or juncture, formed by major cerebral arteries at the base of the brain. Aneurysms are dangerous
because they may place pressure on critical brain areas and rupture, causing subarachnoid hemorrhage. The signs and symptoms
of this disorder depend on what brain area is affected by aneurysmal pressure or rupture.

### Assessment

#### Frequently encountered subjective data
• headache
• intermittent nausea
• irritability
• visual disturbances

#### Frequently encountered objective data
• caused by aneurysmal pressure
    —unilateral hearing loss
    —unilateral dilated pupil
    —inability to rotate eye
    —ptosis
• caused by aneurysmal rupture
    —altered level of consciousness
    —seizures
    —meningeal signs

### Nursing Diagnosis

Altered Tissue Perfusion: Cerebral: Decreased Physiologic-Behavioral Responsiveness related to cerebral ischemia secondary to
increased intracranial pressure (ICP).
*Desired outcome:* The patient will have no signs or symptoms of
increased ICP. If these do occur, they will be recognized and reported promptly.

### Interventions and rationales

1. Take the following aneurysm precautions:
• Enforce complete bed rest.
• Provide subdued lighting.
• Position the head of the bed as ordered.
• Provide a quiet environment.
• Keep emergency equipment available.
• Limit visitors.
• Make sure the patient avoids coffee and stimulants.
*Rationale:* These precautions decrease stress and agitation that can result in hemorrhage, bleeding recurrence, or increased ICP.
2. Monitor the patient for:
• change in level of consciousness or orientation
• bradycardia
• widening pulse pressure
• size, shape, equality, and reaction of pupils
• any neurologic changes or deficits by performing neurologic checks at least every hour.
*Rationale:* Monitoring helps detect early indications of increasing ICP.

## Nursing Diagnosis

Potential Injury: Trauma related to seizures.
*Desired outcome:* The patient's seizures will be prevented or controlled and his safety will be maintained.

### Interventions and rationales

Take the following seizure precautions:
• Keep a *soft* oral airway (or rolled washcloth) at the bedside or taped to the headboard.
• Have emergency medications, such as diazepam, phenytoin, and phenobarbital, readily accessible.
• Provide a quiet atmosphere.
• Provide subdued lighting.
• Avoid nonessential procedures.
• Pad bed rails; keep bed rails up when the patient is in bed.
• Enforce bedrest, if ordered.
• Do not permit unsupervised smoking.
• Do not take oral temperature with glass thermometers.
*Rationale:* These precautions provide for the patient's safety and decrease activity that may stimulate seizures.

## Nursing Diagnosis

Knowledge Deficit related to aneurysm and aneurysm precautions.
*Desired outcome:* The patient can explain what an aneurysm is as well as its potential hazards and can state the rationale for seizure precautions.

## Interventions and rationales

1. Explain what an aneurysm is and the potential threat of rupture. Describe signs and symptoms of an impending rupture. *Rationale:* This promotes compliance with the management routine.

2. Explain aneurysm precautions. *Rationale:* The patient may feel well and not understand the need for precautions and thus may not obey nursing orders.

## Medical Diagnosis

**CT scan** can reveal blood in the subarachnoid space, ventricles, or brain tissue from leak or rupture of cerebral vessel.

**Lumbar puncture** may show red blood cells in the CSF.

**Arteriography,** the definitive test, shows the unruptured cerebral vessel on fluoroscopy.

### Medical treatment

**Codeine** or other analgesics are given for pain or headache as needed. (Use extreme caution if administering opiates or sedatives.)

**Antihypertensives** are administered to maintain normal blood pressure.

**Corticosteroids** are given to prevent edema.

**Phenobarbital** is administered to reduce the seizure threshold.

**Aminocaproic acid** is given to reduce the chance of bleeding recurrences.

**Surgery** may be of benefit.

---

**FAMILY COPING**   **CEREBRAL ANEURYSM**

*Whenever possible, actively involve the patient and family or significant other in discussing:*

• what causes a cerebral aneurysm and how it develops
• aneurysm precautions—activities and behaviors that place the patient at a higher risk for developing increased intracranial pressure, aneurysmal rupture, and dissection
• signs and symptoms that should be reported immediately: syncope, severe headache, blurred vision, as well as numbness, tingling, paralysis, or weakness in an extremity
• medications—actions, side effects, and administration
• diagnostic tests—the purpose, procedure, and how to obtain the results
• surgery, if scheduled.

## ☐ Brain Abscess

A brain abscess is a free or encapsulated collection of pus in the brain. A relatively rare disorder, it is most common in persons age 10 to 35. The infection may start by direct extension of a localized infection, such as a sinus or ear infection, or from bacteremia (systemic blood infection). Signs and symptoms vary with the position of the abscess. The clinical presentation of brain abscess is very similar to that of a tumor because both result from a space-occupying lesion within the cranial vault.

### Assessment

#### Frequently encountered subjective data
• headache (worsened by straining)
• nausea
• visual disturbances
• dizziness

#### Frequently encountered objective data
• changes in level of consciousness (drowsiness or stupor)
• vomiting
• seizures
• nystagmus
• receptive or expressive aphasia
• facial weakness
• tremor
• ataxia
• pupil inequality
• increased ICP

### Nursing Diagnosis

Ineffective Breathing Pattern related to brain stem compression. *Desired outcome:* The patient's normal respiratory rate and pattern will be maintained. Blood gas levels will stay within normal limits. Signs and symptoms of hypoxia will be absent.

#### Interventions and rationales

1. Monitor respiratory rate and pattern, arterial blood gas (ABG) levels, breath sounds, and chest X-rays.
*Rationale:* Such measures ensure early detection of Cheyne-Stokes breathing (see *Abnormal Breathing Patterns Associated with Brain Injury,* page 3) or other abnormal breathing patterns as well as hypoxia from increased ICP. ABG levels are the best indicators of the patient's respiratory status. Normal ranges for ABG levels are $PaO_2$ between 80 and 100 mm Hg, $PaCO_2$ between 35 and 45 mm Hg, and pH between 7.35 and 7.45. ($PaO_2$ <50 mm Hg or $PaCO_2$ >50 mm Hg indicates respiratory failure,

which requires medical intervention).

2. Change the patient's position at least every 2 hours and encourage deep breathing. Discourage frequent or vigorous coughing.
*Rationale:* Shallow breathing and abnormal breathing patterns contribute to stasis and infection. Deep breathing mobilizes secretions, preventing this. Retained secretions increase $PaCO_2$ levels and thus contribute to increased ICP. Coughing increases ICP and is contraindicated.

## Nursing Diagnosis

Potential Injury: Trauma related to loss of motor control secondary to seizures.
*Desired outcome:* Seizures will be prevented, or if they occur, they will be treated promptly with no resulting patient injury.

### Interventions and rationales

Take the following seizure precautions:
• Enforce bed rest, if ordered.
• Keep side rails up at all times; pad rails for safety.
• Keep a soft oral airway (or a rolled washcloth) at the patient's bedside.
• Prohibit unsupervised smoking.
• Do not take oral temperature with glass thermometers.
• Have emergency medications, such as diazepam, phenytoin, and phenobarbital, readily accessible.
*Rationale:* These precautions reduce the chances of spontaneous seizure activity brought about by environmental stimuli and provide for patient safety.

## Nursing Diagnosis

Altered Tissue Perfusion: Cerebral: Decreased Physiologic-Behavioral Responsiveness related to increased ICP.
*Desired outcome:* No signs or symptoms of increased ICP will appear. Neurologic status and vital signs will remain stable. If ICP rises, it will be recognized and reported promptly.

### Interventions and rationales

1. Monitor the patient closely for:
• change in his level of consciousness or orientation
• bradycardia
• widening pulse pressure
• sudden neurologic changes (sensory or motor).
*Rationale:* These signs can indicate increasing ICP.
2. Notify the doctor if you detect:
• sudden loss of consciousness
• pupil dilation or inappropriate response to light
• sudden, pronounced changes in vital signs

• sudden onset of gross neurologic deficit
 —hemiparesis (weakness on one side of the body)
 —hemiplegia (paralysis of one side of the body)
 —facial paralysis, slurred speech
 —aphasia
• abnormal posturing in coma
• abnormal breathing pattern, such as Cheyne-Stokes breathing.
3. Limit fluids unless contraindicated. Keep all I.V. solutions on drip regulators.
*Rationale:* These measures decrease cerebral edema.
4. Monitor intake and output closely.
*Rationale:* Fluid overload may result in increased ICP.

## Medical Diagnosis

**Skull X-rays** can check for possible sources of parameningeal infection. Some abscesses caused by sinusitis occur adjacent to the infected sinus.

**CT scan** with contrast enhancement reveals a typical "doughnut" lesion (a ring surrounding the abscess).

**Arteriography** is used to differentiate a tumor from an abscess when the diagnosis from the CT scan is not clear.

### Medical treatment

**Antibiotics** are given to combat the underlying infection.

**Surgery** can be performed to aspirate or drain the abscess.

**Osmotic diuretics** may be administered to control cerebral edema.

**Glucocorticosteroids** (for example, dexamethasone) can be used to decrease cerebral edema.

**Anticonvulsants** (phenytoin and phenobarbital) are administered to control seizures.

---

**FAMILY COPING** | **BRAIN ABSCESSES**

*Whenever possible, actively involve the patient and family or significant other in discussing:*

• what causes a brain abscess and how it develops
• the signs and symptoms of increased ICP, such as confusion, headache, blurred vision, and syncope, and how to avoid activities that may increase ICP
• the importance of seizure precautions
• diagnostic tests—the purpose, procedure, and how to obtain the results
• medications—actions, side effects, and administration.

# ☐ Cerebrovascular Accident

A cerebrovascular accident (CVA) occurs when the blood supply to a portion of the brain is temporarily interrupted. This interruption can result from occlusion of a cerebral blood vessel (by a clot or thrombus), hemorrhage of a cerebral vessel, or vessel spasm and occlusion from atherosclerotic disease. The consequences of vascular insufficiency are ischemia, and sometimes necrosis, of brain tissue supplied by the affected vessels. The neurologic deficits caused by CVA result directly from the damaged brain tissue. Signs and symptoms of CVA vary with the brain area affected.

## Assessment

### Frequently encountered subjective data

- headache (from hemorrhage), usually of sudden onset
- nausea
- syncope
- tinnitus (ringing or buzzing in the ears)
- muscle weakness (unilateral or bilateral)
- sensory or motor loss
- hemianopia (defective vision or blindness in half of the visual field)
- dysphagia (difficulty swallowing)
- numbness
- complaints of bowel or bladder incontinence

### Frequently encountered objective data

- stupor
- hemiplegia (paralysis on one side of the body)
- hemiparesis (muscle weakness on one side of the body)
- mental confusion
- drooping of the mouth
- generalized muscle weakness
- speech deficit
- paralysis involving face or any extremity

## TRANSIENT ISCHEMIC ATTACKS

Transient ischemic attacks (TIAs) are temporary neurologic deficits that resolve within 24 hours of onset. Patients are assessed to decide if they would benefit from carotid surgery. Arteriography is often performed to check for a correctable carotid artery lesion.

Nonsurgical candidates are given anticoagulant therapy (heparin, then warfarin sodium), if not contraindicated. An alternative regimen is the use of aspirin initially or after 3 months of warfarin therapy.

Nursing care of the TIA patient involves close monitoring of vital signs and periodic neurologic checks to detect further neurologic deficits that may indicate stroke-in-evolution (developing stroke). Nursing diagnoses are made based on assessment of the patient's needs and neurologic deficits, as in cerebrovascular accident.

- aphasia (receptive or expressive)
- flushed face
- bowel or bladder incontinence
- personality changes
- seizures
- coma
- unequal or fixed pupil(s)
- nystagmus (rapid eye movement toward and away from midline)
- deviation of eyes toward the side of the lesion (cerebellar hemorrhage)
- meningeal signs (see page 63)

## Nursing Diagnosis

Alterations in Tissue Perfusion: Cerebral: Decreased Behavioral Responsiveness and Sensory-Motor Impairment related to cerebral ischemia.
*Desired outcome:* The patient's brain perfusion and cerebral blood flow will be maintained. Body cells and tissues will be adequately oxygenated.

### Interventions and rationales

1. Assess the patient for change in level of consciousness. Perform neurologic checks every 2 hours or as often as indicated by patient instability.
*Rationale:* Ischemic brain tissue can become edematous, causing a rise in ICP. Frequently, a change in level of consciousness is the first sign of increased ICP.
2. Measure vital signs every 2 hours or more frequently if needed. Observe for widening pulse pressure and decreased heart rate.
*Rationale:* These vital signs may indicate increased ICP.
3. Monitor intake and output, ABG measurements, urine specific gravity, and blood pressure.
*Rationale:* Dehydration must be recognized early because hemoconcentration and decreased blood volume result in decreased cerebral blood flow. Signs and symptoms of dehydration usually include dry skin and mucous membranes, increased urine specific gravity (>1.020), decreased urine output, and decreased blood pressure.

## Nursing Diagnosis

Impaired Physical Mobility related to hemiplegia or hemiparesis.
*Desired outcome:* The patient will understand and practice self-care activities taught by the nurse. Mobility will be maintained at a recorded optimal level.

## Interventions and rationales

1. Provide range-of-motion exercises to all extremities every 8 hours.
*Rationale:* This helps prevent muscle contractures and loss of muscle tone.
2. Observe for and record changes in weakness or paralysis.
*Rationale:* This helps determine progressive neurologic recovery or deterioration.
3. Maintain the affected extremities in functional positions using splints. Elevate the extremities higher than the heart level.
*Rationale:* This prevents contractures and dependent edema.
4. When the patient is supine, support the affected hip and thigh with a trochanter roll.
*Rationale:* This prevents external rotation of leg.
5. Teach the patient progressive isometric exercises when possible.
*Rationale:* This improves muscle tone.
6. Turn the patient every 2 hours to his back and unaffected side.
*Rationale:* This prevents or minimizes edema and improves pulmonary drainage.
7. Teach the patient how to turn from side to side using a trapeze or side rails.
*Rationale:* This promotes independent function and prevents hip contractures.
8. When his vital signs are stable, prepare the patient to sit:
• Place the affected arm across the chest.
• Using his normal arm, have the patient fold the affected leg over the normal leg.
• Have the patient position himself on the edge of the bed, pushing against the mattress with the unaffected arm.
• When the patient is sitting, adjust the affected arm and leg with the normal arm and leg.
*Rationale:* Resuming activity as soon as the patient can tolerate it helps restore optimal function.

## Nursing Diagnosis

Impaired Verbal Communication related to aphasia.
*Desired outcome:* The patient will understand and practice methods of facilitating communication taught by the nurse. Communication will be maintained.

### Interventions and rationales

1. Assess the type and severity of aphasia:
• receptive aphasia
    —auditory aphasia: Does the patient hear words?
    —visual aphasia: Does the patient understand written language?
    —motor alexia: Does the patient have trouble reading aloud?
• expressive aphasia
    —motor aphasia: Does the patient have difficulty expressing
      thoughts in speech or writing?

## DIFFERENTIATING BETWEEN COMMUNICATION DISORDERS

| Disorder | Clinical findings | Location of lesion |
|----------|-------------------|--------------------|
| Broca's aphasia (motor expressive nonfluent) | Patient knows what he wants to say, but has motor impairment and can't articulate spontaneously. Also, patient understands written or verbal requests but can't repeat words or phrases. | Frontal (posterior) |
| Wernicke's aphasia (sensory receptive/expressive fluent) | Patient articulates spontaneously and well, but uses words inappropriately or uses neologisms. Also, patient has difficulty understanding written or verbal requests and can't repeat words or phrases. | Temporoparietal (anterior) |
| Global aphasia | Patient has profound expressive and receptive deficits and can barely communicate. | Temporoparietal |
| Anomia | When given an object, patient can describe its characteristics (color, size, purpose) but cannot name it. | Parietal, subcortical, or temporal |
| Apraxia | When asked to speak, patient can't coordinate movement of lips and tongue. When left alone, he may be able to do so. | Frontal |
| Dysarthria | Patient knows what he wants to say, but has motor impairment and fails to speak clearly. Also, patient has difficulty swallowing and chewing. | Cerebellar or frontal (posterior) |
| Perseveration | Patient continually repeats one idea or response. | Throughout cerebrum (primarily anterior) |

—agraphia: Does the patient have difficulty writing?

—dysarthria: Does the patient have slurred speech?

—mixed aphasia: Does the patient exhibit any combination of any of the above groups?

*Rationale:* This establishes a baseline of expression and comprehension ability.

2. Talk directly to the patient, slowly and distinctly, and communicate from his unaffected side.

*Rationale:* Although the patient's response may be absent or distorted, direct communication contributes to the patient's self-concept.

3. Provide alternative methods of communication, such as aphasia boards, picture cards, paper and pencil, or hand gestures, to assist in expression.

*Rationale:* An aphasia board is a communication aid that can be adapted to the patient's needs. It promotes independence and reduces patient frustration.

4. Encourage speech by repeating words slowly and by asking questions that require one-word answers. Consult a speech therapist.

*Rationale:* This reinforces communication skills and allows patient to practice frequently used words and phrases.

## Nursing Diagnosis

Altered Nutrition: Less than Body Requirements: Decreased Intake related to paralysis or altered level of consciousness.

*Desired outcome:* The patient's nutritional balance will be maintained. A minimum daily caloric intake of (specify caloric amount) will be ingested by the patient.

### Interventions and rationales

1. Assess the patient for dysphagia and the inability to feed himself. Adjust food and nursing care to the patient's ability to eat and drink by providing finger foods and assistive devices.

*Rationale:* This gives the patient a sense of independence and increases his self-esteem. Independence offers the patient a chance to select foods from his plate and eat at his own pace. This provides additional motivation to complete meals.

2. Maintain balanced intake and output and record on bedside flowsheet.

*Rationale:* Fluids are monitored to prevent dehydration, a common complication of CVA, especially in elderly persons.

3. Increase the diet's texture as tolerated.

*Rationale:* This will increase the patient's ability to feed himself progressively.

## Nursing Diagnosis

Sensory-Perceptual Alterations: Decreased Sensory Acuity (specify visual, auditory, gustatory, tactile, kinesthetic, or olfactory) related to central nervous system changes secondary to CVA.

*Desired outcome:* Patient will function to the extent of his capabilities in an environment temporarily modified by the nurse.

### Interventions and rationales

1. Assess the patient for sensory awareness. Does he recognize sensations of heat and cold, or dullness and sharpness? Is he aware of motion and location of body parts? Does he have a restricted field of vision?

*Rationale:* The nurse can provide for patient safety.

2. Arrange the patient's personal articles, call bell, and food trays on his unaffected side.

*Rationale:* This helps take advantage of the patient's functional sensory and motor capacities.

3. Identify positions of affected body areas when moving the patient.

*Rationale:* The patient may have lost the ability to spatially perceive body positions.

4. Keep side rails up at all times.

*Rationale:* This ensures patient safety.

5. Examine the patient's eyes for irritation and inflammation. Cleanse and lubricate the eyes as needed.

*Rationale:* The corneal reflex may be absent, causing the eyes to dry out (since no blinking occurs).

6. Maintain optimum body alignment by using a footboard or splint, placing a pillow under the affected axilla to prevent adduction, or using trochanter rolls to prevent external rotation of legs.

*Rationale:* The patient may not be able to perceive position or pain in an extremity. Alignment maintains the functional position of the extremities and prevents muscle contractures.

### Nursing Diagnosis

Self-Care Deficit (specify bathing/hygiene, dressing/grooming, toileting, or feeding) related to sensory or motor impairment.

*Desired outcome:* The patient will remain motivated toward rehabilitation. The patient will perform activities of daily living that are within his ability, using acquired techniques and assistive equipment.

### Interventions and rationales

1. Assess the extent of the patient's ability to feed self, bathe, dress, toilet, and maintain hygiene.

*Rationale:* This establishes the patient's need for assistance or assistive devices.

2. Avoid doing anything for the patient that he can do for himself.

*Rationale:* This discourages dependence.

3. Be consistently supportive, yet firm.
*Rationale:* Consistency develops trust in the nurse-patient relationship and improves patient cooperation.
4. Provide self-help devices as needed.
*Rationale:* This encourages independence and discourages frustration.
5. Assist the patient to the bathroom every 2 hours for voiding.
*Rationale:* The patient may be unable to communicate his elimination needs.
6. Identify normal bowel habits and establish a bowel regimen.
*Rationale:* This aids in bowel retraining.
7. Provide dietary bulk and ensure sufficient fluid intake.
*Rationale:* This helps prevent constipation.

## Nursing Diagnosis
Dysfunctional Grieving: Depression related to loss of self-esteem, loss of body function, and decreased self-image.
*Desired outcome:* The patient will cooperate with rehabilitative activities and show no signs of clinical depression.

### Interventions and rationales
1. Assess the patient's ability to comprehend the spoken word. Can he follow directions? Are his responses appropriate?
*Rationale:* Neurologic deficits may be subtle; the patient's judgment and intellectual ability may be impaired by brain damage. Pay special attention to the patient's affect and the appropriateness of his responses. Therapeutic interventions related to depression are not effective unless you are familiar with the patient's functional level of comprehension.
2. Take a thorough social history to determine previous occupational activities and hobbies.
*Rationale:* The patient may be able to resume certain aspects of his career or hobbies; he may need counseling to adjust to permanent neurologic deficits.
3. Explain all nursing procedures.
*Rationale:* This allows the patient to assist when possible and helps relieve anxiety and decrease feelings of uselessness.
4. Assign the patient to the same personnel when possible.
*Rationale:* This helps establish a trusting environment and encourages the patient to communicate his feelings.

## Nursing Diagnosis
Impaired Gas Exchange and Ineffective Breathing Pattern related to neurologic deficit.
*Desired outcome:* The patient's airway will remain unobstructed, and adequate ventilation will be maintained. Pathologic breathing patterns will be recognized and reported.

## Interventions and rationales

1. Observe the patient for slow or rapid respiratory rate, change in respiratory pattern, cyanosis, and other physical signs of hypoxia.
*Rationale:* These observations will reflect signs and symptoms of respiratory difficulty or depression caused by neurologic damage.
2. Monitor ABG measurements.
*Rationale:* Any neurologic deficit that results in altered breathing patterns can produce impaired gas exchange that may progress to respiratory failure ($PaO_2$ < 50 mm Hg, $PaCO_2$ > 50 mm Hg).

## Nursing Diagnosis

Potential for Injury: Trauma related to loss of awareness and motor control secondary to seizures.
*Desired outcome:* The patient will have no seizures while taking anticonvulsant medication. If seizures do occur, patient safety will be maintained.

### Interventions and rationales

Take the following seizure precautions:
• Enforce bed rest, if ordered; pad bed rails and keep them in an upright position while patient is in bed.
• Tape a soft airway (or rolled washcloth) to the headboard.
• Maintain a quiet environment.
• Forbid unsupervised smoking.
• Take no oral temperatures with a glass thermometer.
• Keep emergency anticonvulsant medications, such as I.V. diazepam, phenytoin, and phenobarbital, readily accessible.
*Rationale:* These measures diminish the risk of spontaneous seizure activity brought on by environmental stimuli, thereby providing for patient safety.

## Medical Diagnosis

Medical diagnosis of CVA is based on a thorough medical history and laboratory and diagnostic test results.

**CBC and SMA 12/60** can detect systemic causes of CVA, such as polycythemia or serious anemias.

**CT scan** localizes the lesion and can differentiate hemorrhage from other space-occupying lesions.

**Lumbar puncture** usually reveals elevated CSF pressure and grossly bloody fluid in subarachnoid and intracerebral hemorrhage. In thrombosis, it may show elevated total CSF protein levels.

**EEG** helps locate areas of abnormal brain activity.

**Skull X-rays** may reveal a shifting to the opposite side of an expanding mass. Internal carotid calcifications may be visible on X-ray with thrombosis; partial calcification on an aneurysm's walls also may be detected.

**Cerebral angiography** can detect arterial obstruction and narrowing of the circle of Willis or its branches, arteriovenous malformations, or hemorrhagic areas (seen as avascular zones surrounded by displaced arteries and veins).

## Medical treatment

**Anticonvulsants**, such as diazepam, phenytoin, and phenobarbital, to treat and prevent seizures.

**Stool softeners** to help prevent straining at stool, which increases ICP.

**Analgesics** such as codeine to relieve headache.

**Carotid artery surgery** may be performed in patients with documented carotid artery obstruction.

---

**FAMILY COPING** | **CEREBROVASCULAR ACCIDENTS**

*Whenever possible, actively involve the patient and family or significant other in discussing:*

• how the brain controls motor function and what causes a cerebrovascular accident
• diagnostic tests—the purpose, procedure, and how to obtain the results
• the importance of rehabilitation in reducing neurologic deficits
• dietary adjustments, such as using semisoft foods for dysphagia
• assistive devices and home safety measures
• medications—actions, side effects, and administration
• surgery, if necessary
• local sources of additional help, such as home health care and rehabilitation services.

## ☐ Encephalitis

Encephalitis is a brain inflammation usually caused by a virus. Mumps, enterovirus, herpes simplex, and mosquito-borne and tick-borne viruses are the most common etiologies. The virus causes an intense lymphocytic infiltration of brain tissue and the meninges, resulting in cerebral edema, degeneration of ganglion cells, and diffuse nervous tissue dysfunction.

## Assessment

### Frequently encountered subjective data
• headache
• drowsiness
• nausea

### Frequently encountered objective data
• fever
• change in level of consciousness
—lethargy to coma
—disorientation

• meningeal signs (see page 63)
• seizures
• ataxia (lack of coordination)
• vomiting

## Nursing Diagnosis

Altered Tissue Perfusion: Cerebral: Decreased Physiologic-Behavioral Responsiveness related to increased ICP.
*Desired outcome:* Patient will have no signs or symptoms of increased ICP. If signs and symptoms do occur, they will be recognized and reported promptly.

### Interventions and rationales

1. Monitor the patient closely for:
• change in level of consciousness or orientation
• bradycardia
• widening pulse pressure
• sudden behaviorial changes or sensory and motor deficits.
*Rationale:* All can be signs of increasing ICP.
2. Notify the doctor of the following signs and symptoms:
• pupil that becomes dilated or does not respond appropriately to light
• sudden loss of consciousness
• sudden pronounced changes in vital signs, such as bradycardia or widening pulse pressure
• sudden onset of gross neurologic deficits
    — hemiparesis
    — hemiplegia
    — facial paralysis
    — slurred speech
    — aphasia
• onset of abnormal posturing in coma (see page 16)
• abnormal breathing pattern, such as Cheyne-Stokes breathing.
*Rationale:* These ominous signs of brain stem compression or herniation require a neurosurgeon's immediate attention.
3. Limit fluids if not contraindicated.
*Rationale:* This helps to decrease cerebral edema.

## Nursing Diagnosis

Potential Impaired Skin Integrity related to immobility.
*Desired outcome:* No signs of skin breakdown (redness, blistering, necrosis, open areas, petechiae, or tissue thinness) will occur.

### Interventions and rationales

1. Examine the patient's skin (especially bony prominences) for reddened areas every 8 hours.
*Rationale:* Redness is the first sign of skin inflammation and impending breakdown.

2. Keep the patient's skin dry.
*Rationale:* Moisture encourages bacterial growth and may lead to infection of damaged skin.
3. Massage around bony prominences.
*Rationale:* This increases circulation and helps prevent ischemic breakdown.
4. Pad bony prominences whenever possible.
*Rationale:* This helps distribute weight around bony areas.
5. Place the patient on a flotation or alternating-pressure mattress or on a turning frame. Change his position at least every 2 hours; do not position on affected areas.
*Rationale:* This helps alternate weight distribution and increases circulation by keeping pressure off bony prominences for extended periods.

## Nursing Diagnosis
Impaired Gas Exchange related to immobility.
*Desired outcome:* No signs or symptoms of atelectasis or impaired gas exchange will occur.

### Interventions and rationales
1. Auscultate the patient's breath sounds every 2 hours.
*Rationale:* You are observing breath sounds for crackles, rhonchi, or diminished sounds on auscultation that indicate congestion or consolidation of lung tissue.
2. Change the patient's position every 2 hours.
*Rationale:* This helps mobilize secretions and aerate lung sections compromised by positioning.
3. Encourage coughing and deep breathing, if not contraindicated by increased ICP.
*Rationale:* This helps mobilize secretions to be expelled.
4. Perform nasotracheal suctioning when you detect lung congestion (indicated by coarse crackles or rhonchi). Check with the doctor before suctioning; it may be contraindicated.
*Rationale:* This clears the major airways to permit better gas exchange.
5. Monitor ABG levels.
*Rationale:* This helps you evaluate the adequacy of ventilation. Normal levels are: $PaO_2$ from 80 to 100 mm Hg, $PaCO_2$ from 35 to 45 mm Hg, and pH from 7.35 to 7.45.

## Nursing Diagnosis
Potential Impaired Physical Mobility related to muscle contractures.
*Desired outcome:* No contractures will occur.

### Interventions and rationales
1. Provide range-of-motion exercises to all extremities every 8 hours.

*Rationale:* This stretches joint muscles, maintaining flexibility.

2. Maintain proper body alignment.

*Rationale:* This keeps muscles and joints in a functional position.

3. Use splints for the patient's affected wrists and feet (see page 101). Do not use splints on extremities that are dependent when patient is turned.

*Rationale:* This prevents wrist contractures and footdrop and keeps hands and feet in a functional position. Splints are rigid and can cause tissue damage if they are under patient when turned.

## Nursing Diagnosis

Potential for Physical Injury: Trauma related to altered level of consciousness.

*Desired outcome:* Patient safety will be maintained.

### Interventions and rationales

1. Keep side rails up.

*Rationale:* This helps prevent injury if the patient becomes disoriented or has a seizure.

2. Remove dentures, contact lenses, and other prostheses until the patient regains full consciousness.

*Rationale:* This helps prevent injury to gums, corneas, and skin from prolonged contact with the prosthesis.

3. Examine the patient's eyes frequently for irritation and inflammation that may occur from decreased tearing and the inability to moisten eyes by blinking. Lubricating drops should be administered prophylactically.

*Rationale:* This prevents corneal ulceration.

4. Take seizure precautions. (See pages 116 to 117.)

*Rationale:* This provides for patient safety in the event of a seizure.

## Medical Diagnosis

**Lumbar puncture** identifies the virus in CSF, confirming the diagnosis. It also reveals elevated CSF pressure.

**EEG** is usually abnormal with encephalitis.

**CT scan** can rule out hematoma.

**Brain biopsy** can identify a treatable viral infection, such as herpes.

### Medical treatment

**Vidarabine and acyclovir** are effective against herpes encephalitis.

Treatment of all other forms of encephalitis is **supportive**, involving dilantin and other anticonvulsants, glucocorticosteroids to decrease cerebral edema, sedatives to reduce restlessness, aspirin to reduce fever, and I.V. fluid therapy to ensure electrolyte and fluid balance.

| FAMILY COPING | ENCEPHALITIS |
| --- | --- |

*Whenever possible, actively involve the patient and family or significant other in discussing:*

• how the disease causes swelling and brain cell damage and the resulting signs and symptoms
• diagnostic tests—the purpose, procedure, and how to obtain results
• I.V. therapy and medications
• monitoring and life support equipment in use
• the importance of seizure precautions.

# ☐ Epilepsy

Epilepsy is a brain condition that renders the patient susceptible to seizures. Seizures may occur spontaneously or may follow an aura. For more about seizures and their management, see pages 115 to 120.

## Assessment

### Frequently encountered subjective data
• blackouts
• incontinence after an unconscious period
• amnesic episodes
• mental disturbances
• muscle tremors
• spastic muscle movement
• hallucinations

### Frequently encountered objective data
• recurrent episodes of unconsciousness with tonic-clonic jerking (may be elicited by loud noises, music, flickering lights, or exhaustion)
• apparent lapses or alterations in consciousness

## Nursing Diagnosis

Potential for Injury: Trauma related to lack of awareness and lack of motor control secondary to recurrent seizure activity.
*Desired outcome:* The patient's seizures will be controlled by anticonvulsant medications. Patient safety will be maintained in the event of a seizure.

### Interventions and rationales
1. Take the following seizure precautions:
• Enforce strict bed rest if ordered.
• Allow bathroom privileges, with assistance.
• Pad side rails and keep them up while patient is in bed.

• Keep a soft oral airway or a rolled washcloth at the bedside to insert before an impending seizure.
• Forbid unsupervised smoking.
• Take no oral temperatures with glass thermometers.
• Keep emergency anticonvulsant medications, such as I.V. diazepam, phenytoin, and phenobarbital, readily available.
*Rationale:* The patient may become restless immediately before a seizure. A rubber oral airway or rolled washcloth inserted in the mouth during an aura, or preseizure experience, or a restless period can prevent tongue biting and airway occlusion by the tongue when the seizure occurs. Do not use rigid plastic airways; they will damage teeth, which may result in aspiration of tooth fragments. Do not attempt to insert the airway while the patient is having a seizure. Bed rest, bathroom privileges, and side rails are for the patient's protection. Seizures may occur at any time, apparently without warning; do not use glass thermometers for oral temperatures.
2. Observe and record characteristics of an aura, if present.
*Rationale:* This allows for planning and patient teaching. If the patient recognizes periods that precede seizure activity, he can seek help. This also may help the patient to identify and avoid specific factors that precipitate a seizure.
3. Observe and record seizure activity.
• Before the seizure (preictal stage), check for:
  —level of consciousness
  —activity before attack
  —portion of the body in which the seizure started.
• During the seizure (interictal stage), check for:
  —the patient crying out
  —automatisms, such as eye fluttering or lip smacking
  —bilateral movements
  —length of the seizure
  —salivation
  —cyanosis
  —incontinence
  —pupil activity.
• After the seizure (postictal stage), check for:
  —lethargy
  —confusion
  —headache
  —speech impairment
  —other neurologic deficits, such as transient hemiplegia.
*Rationale:* Careful observation helps the doctor in diagnosing the location and time of seizure activity.
4. Intervene appropriately, as follows:
• Support the patient's head.
• Lower the patient to the floor if he is standing at the seizure's onset.

• Insert a soft oral airway or rolled washcloth if the full onset of the seizure has not occurred yet.
• Maintain adequate airway and oxygenation to whatever extent is possible.
• Observe and report the event according to the above observation criteria.
• Give medication as ordered.
• Reorient the patient after the seizure.
*Rationale:* Appropriate nursing interventions protect the patient from injury.
5. Observe for side effects and effectiveness of medications (for further information on the following or other anticonvulsants, see Section 7):
• I.V. diazepam (Valium) used as a muscle relaxant or an anticonvulsant has several adverse effects, including ataxia, dizziness, slurred speech, tremors, hypotension, bradycardia, and cardiovascular collapse (shock). Diazepam also potentiates phenobarbital.
• Phenobarbital (Luminal) used as an anticonvulsant or a sedative has several adverse effects, including central nervous system (CNS) depression, drowsiness, lethargy, and stupor. You should monitor the patient closely for potentiated CNS depression when giving this drug with diazepam.
• Phenytoin (Dilantin), an anticonvulsant, has several adverse effects, including thrombocytopenia (decreased number of blood platelets), leukopenia (a deficient number of leukocytes), hypotension, and ventricular irritability (dysrhythmias or irregular pulse).
*Rationale:* By observing for possible adverse effects of medications, you can help maintain the patient's safety. An accurate record of seizure progression and response to medication is of diagnostic value. Your observations may help the doctor in locating the area of brain irritability.

## Nursing Diagnosis
Knowledge Deficit related to disease management.
*Desired outcome:* The patient will verbalize the nature of his seizure disorder, as well as precautions and the treatment regimen.

### Interventions and rationales
1. Discuss the patient's feelings and fears about epilepsy, and correct any misconceptions.
*Rationale:* This helps dispel unjustified fears and eliminates misinformation.
2. Discuss his medications and their side effects as well as the consequences of noncompliance and situations that may necessitate a change in dosage.
*Rationale:* This encourages strict adherence to the medication regimen.

3. Obtain a Medic Alert tag for the patient and instruct him to wear it at all times.
*Rationale:* This ensures diagnostic identification by medical personnel.

## Medical Diagnosis

**EEG** may help locate the area of cerebral malfunction.

**Telemetry monitoring** monitors the brain's electrical activity, helping to identify the prodromal period so that seizures can be predicted and controlled.

**Skull X-rays** can rule out injury or a space-occupying lesion.

**Lumbar puncture** can rule out infection and increased ICP.

**CT scan** can rule out a space-occupying lesion not found on X-ray.

## Medical treatment

Commonly prescribed **anticonvulsants** include carbamazepine, clonazepam, ethosuximide, phenobarbital, phenytoin, primidone, and valproic acid. (For more about seizure management, see pages 116 to 120.)

---

**FAMILY COPING | EPILEPSY**

*Whenever possible, actively involve the patient and family or significant other in discussing:*

• how irritable brain tissue can cause electrical activity that results in a seizure
• factors that may trigger a seizure, such as fatigue and hypoglycemia
• diagnostic tests—the purpose, procedure, and how to obtain the results
• the importance of seizure precautions and wearing a Medic Alert bracelet or pendant
• how the family or significant other should observe and care for the patient during a seizure
• medications—actions, side effects, and administration.

## ☐ Guillain-Barré Syndrome

Guillain-Barré syndrome is a form of polyneuritis (nerve inflammation) that results in a rapidly progressive, and sometimes even fatal, muscle weakness. Patients also suffer distal sensory loss. Although about 95% of the patients recover spontaneously, some may have persistent mild motor deficits. If symptoms continue longer than 20 days after onset, the prognosis is poor. Symptoms develop in an ascending order: legs are affected first, then the trunk, arms, and finally the CNS.

## Assessment
### Frequently encountered subjective data
• extreme weakness
• numbness or pain in lower extremities
• paresthesia (abnormal burning or tingling sensations)
• difficulty breathing
### Frequently encountered objective data
• extreme muscle weakness (ascending)
• facial diplegia (paralysis of similar areas on both sides of body)
• dysarthria
• hypotonia
• areflexia
• flaccid quadriplegia
• loss of bowel or bladder control
• respiratory distress

## Nursing Diagnosis
Ineffective Breathing Pattern related to hypoventilation secondary to ascending paralysis of respiratory muscles.
*Desired outcome:* Normal respiratory pattern will be maintained.

### Interventions and rationales
1. Assess respiratory rate and rhythm, breathing pattern, and breath sounds every 2 hours.
*Rationale:* This establishes a baseline of respiratory function, allowing monitoring of progress or deterioration.
2. Observe for ascending sensory loss every hour.
*Rationale:* This type of loss usually precedes motor loss.
3. Take a serial vital capacity recording with a respirometer every 8 hours.
*Rationale:* A vital capacity of 800 ml indicates impending respiratory failure warranting respiratory support.

## Nursing Diagnosis
Ineffective Gas Exchange related to hypoventilation.
*Desired outcome:* ABG levels will be normal.

### Interventions and rationales
1. Monitor ABG levels.
*Rationale:* Neuromuscular disease results in primary hypoventilation. Be alert for increased $PaCO_2$ levels (> 50 mm Hg) and decreased $PaO_2$ levels (< 50 mm Hg), which indicate respiratory failure.
2. Auscultate breath sounds every 2 hours. Encourage coughing and deep breathing. Suction if breath sounds indicate congestion (coarse crackles or rhonchi).

## TESTING FOR THORACIC SENSATION

When Guillain-Barré syndrome progresses rapidly, test for ascending sensory loss by touching the patient or pressing his skin lightly with a pin every hour. Move systematically from the iliac crest (T12) to the scapula, occasionally substituting the blunt end of the pin to test the patient's ability to discriminate between sharp and dull. Mark the level of diminished sensation to measure any change. If diminished sensation ascends to T8 or higher, the patient's intercostal muscle function (and consequently respiratory function) will probably be impaired. As Guillain-Barré syndrome subsides, sensory and motor weakness descends to the lower thoracic segments, heralding a return of intercostal and extremity muscle function.

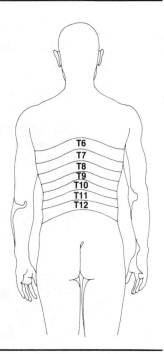

*Rationale:* The airway must be kept clear for adequate gas exchange.

3. Establish an emergency airway if respiratory failure is imminent (this should be done by trained personnel only).

*Rationale:* Mechanical ventilation will be required if respiratory failure occurs. You may want to have emergency airway equipment on hand; if not, be sure you know where to locate it in your area.

## Nursing Diagnosis

Impaired Physical Mobility related to ascending paralysis.

*Desired outcome:* No signs or symptoms of contracture (such as pain, joint stiffness, or deformity) will occur.

### Interventions and rationales

1. Maintain extremities in functional positions, using rolled towels or splints.

*Rationale:* When muscle innervation is lost, flexor muscles have no opposition, resulting in functional positioning loss.

2. Provide range-of-motion exercises to all extremities every 8 hours.

*Rationale:* This keeps joints flexible.

3. Provide for correct body alignment.

*Rationale:* This prevents disabling contractures, especially of the hip, shoulder, and foot.

## Nursing Diagnosis

Impaired Skin Integrity related to immobility.
*Desired outcome:* No signs or symptoms of ischemic skin break-down (pain, redness, blistering, necrosis, petechiae, or tissue thinness) will occur.

### Interventions and rationales

1. Examine the patient's skin (especially bony prominences) for reddened areas at least once every 8 hours.
*Rationale:* Redness is the first sign of inflammation and skin breakdown.
2. Keep the patient's skin dry.
*Rationale:* Moisture encourages bacterial growth and infection of damaged skin.
3. Massage around bony prominences.
*Rationale:* This increases circulation and prevents ischemic breakdown.
4. Place the patient on a flotation or alternating-pressure mattress or on a turning frame. Change the patient's position at least every 2 hours, keeping off affected areas.
*Rationale:* This helps alternate weight distribution and keeps weight off bony prominences.

## Nursing Diagnosis

Altered Nutrition: Less than Body Requirements: Decreased In-take related to dysphagia or inability to feed self.
*Desired outcome:* Normal body weight will be maintained.

### Interventions and rationales

1. Assess the patient's ability to chew and swallow food.
*Rationale:* This serves as a basis for selecting a diet with an appropriate consistency.
2. Assist with feeding to whatever extent is necessary.
*Rationale:* This ensures adequate intake.
3. Keep a suction machine readily accessible if the patient has trouble swallowing or has a fear of choking.
*Rationale:* This provides for patient safety if the patient aspirates food or secretions.

## Medical Diagnosis

**Lumbar puncture** may show an elevated CSF protein level from nerve inflammation. CSF pressure may be elevated in severe cases.

**Electromyography** may show repeated firing of the same motor unit, as opposed to widespread sectional stimulation, and slowed nerve conduction velocities soon after the onset of paralysis.

### Medical treatment

Medical treatment is predominantly supportive, involving intubation and mechanical ventilation if the patient has respiratory problems.

| FAMILY COPING | GUILLAIN-BARRÉ SYNDROME |
| --- | --- |

*Whenever possible, actively involve the patient and family or significant other in discussing:*

• how symptoms develop in ascending order and the progressive nature of neuromuscular impairment
• that 95% of patients recover with little or no impairment
• diagnostic tests—the purpose, procedure, and how to obtain the results
• monitoring and life-support equipment in use.

## ☐ Herniated Intervertebral Disk

Intervertebral disks are fibrocartilaginous pads located between the vertebrae that help make the spine flexible and resilient. The fibrous outer part (anulus fibrosus) surrounds a central gelatinous core (nucleus pulposus). Herniation occurs when trauma or a weakening of the anulus fibrosus causes all or part of the nucleus pulposus to protrude. A major cause of low back pain, a herniated disk may impinge on spinal nerve roots or the spinal cord and produce signs and symptoms of nerve root irritation.

### Assessment

#### Frequently encountered subjective data
• severe low back pain—which sometimes radiates to legs—or neck, arm, or chest pain (symptoms vary, depending on the disk area affected)
• intensified pain with coughing, sneezing, and bending
• numbness or tingling in an extremity

#### Frequently encountered objective data
• sensory or motor loss in areas innervated by a compressed nerve root
• weakness or atrophy of leg muscles
• loss of ankle or knee-jerk reflex

### Nursing Diagnosis

Altered Comfort: Chronic Pain related to nerve root compression.
*Desired outcome:* Pain is relieved or controlled.

#### Interventions and rationales
1. Assess the patient for neurologic deficits.
*Rationale:* Because sensory and motor impairment are signs of

the disorder, assessment helps establish a baseline of neurologic function.

2. Encourage bed rest and changing position from a flat to low Fowler's position to one with a slight knee flex.
*Rationale:* This relieves muscle spasm, prevents or reduces edema, and relieves the stress of body weight on the affected disk.

3. Instruct the patient in relaxation and visualization techniques.
*Rationale:* This helps reduce muscle tension and related pain.

## Nursing Diagnosis
Potential Urinary Retention related to compression of nerves associated with bladder function.
*Desired outcome:* The bladder is emptied at each voiding with no urinary retention.

### Interventions and rationales
1. Record fluid intake and output.
*Rationale:* Prolonged periods between voiding may indicate bladder dysfunction caused by neurologic impairment.

2. Check the bladder for distention every 4 hours.
*Rationale:* Distention signals retention.

3. Report and record incontinence.
*Rationale:* Incontinence indicates loss of sphincter control, possibly from neuromuscular bladder dysfunction.

4. Obtain an order for intermittent catheterization, if necessary.
*Rationale:* Bladder distention on a 4-hour check indicates the need for catheterization.

## Nursing Diagnosis
Impaired Physical Mobility related to pain from muscle spasm associated with nerve compression.
*Desired outcome:* Mobility and muscle tone will be restored and maintained.

### Interventions and rationales
1. Encourage the patient to move his legs (if allowed) or to do isometric leg exercises.
*Rationale:* These activities increase circulation and maintain muscle tone.

2. Splint the patient's ankles, keeping the splints on for 2 hours, then off for 2 hours, if one or both legs are paralyzed.
*Rationale:* Splinting maintains a functional position and prevents footdrop.

## Nursing Diagnosis
Impaired Skin Integrity related to immobility.
*Desired outcome:* No signs of skin breakdown (redness, pain, tissue thinning, petechiae, or necrosis) will occur.

## Interventions and rationales

1. Instruct the patient to avoid sitting and high Fowler's position for prolonged periods. Change his position from flat to low Fowler's every 2 hours while he's in bed (if allowed).
*Rationale:* These measures relieve pressure on the sacral bony prominence.
2. Massage around the patient's sacral prominence, back, and heels while he is lying flat.
*Rationale:* Massage increases circulation in these areas.
3. Keep the patient's skin dry.
*Rationale:* Incontinent patients are at greater risk for skin infection and breakdown from moisture.
4. Encourage adequate fluid intake.
*Rationale:* Fluid intake hydrates skin and helps prevent the breakdown associated with dry skin.

## Medical Diagnosis

**Myelography** may show evidence of disk herniation.

**CT scan** helps localize the area of herniation.

**X-rays** can rule out other lesions.

**Lumbar puncture** can rule out other conditions, such as bloody CSF and infection.

**Magnetic resonance imaging (MRI)** may give better resolution of herniated disks than a CT scan.

### Medical treatment
**Pharmacologic management** may involve:
• analgesics
• muscle relaxants
• anti-inflammatory agents
• steroids.
**Surgical management** may include laminectomy to remove the herniated disk and fusion to stabilize the spine.

---

**FAMILY COPING**  |  **HERNIATED DISKS**

*Whenever possible, actively involve the patient and family or significant other in discussing:*

• how the disk impinges on spinal nerve roots, causing pain (using a model of the vertebral column, if available)
• diagnostic tests—the purpose, procedure, and how to obtain the results
• medications—actions, side effects, and administration
• surgery, if indicated.

## ☐ Meningitis

Meningitis is an inflammation of the pia mater and arachnoid membranes that cover the spinal cord. This inflammation can be caused by bacteria, viruses, fungi, chemical agents, or parasites attacking the subarachnoid space. The presentation of meningitis varies. However, certain signs are common to all meningeal inflammations. (See *Meningeal Signs* below.)

## Assessment

### Frequently encountered subjective data

- severe headache
- neck, back, and leg pain
- drowsiness
- fever
- photophobia
- nausea

---

### MENINGEAL SIGNS

**Testing for Brudzinski's sign**

Place your patient in the dorsal recumbent position, putting your hands behind her neck and bending it forward. The sign's *positive* if pain and resistance are present and if the patient flexes her hips and knees in response to the maneuver.

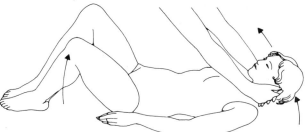

**Testing for Kernig's sign**

With your patient supine, flex her leg at the hip and knee, then try to straighten her knee. The sign's *positive* if pain and resistance are present.

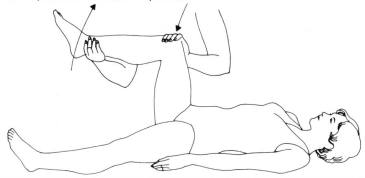

### Frequently encountered objective data
• anorexia
• seizures
• disorientation or delirium
• meningeal signs
   —nuchal rigidity (resistance to forward neck flexion)
   —fever and chills (with infection)
   —increased sensitivity to light
   —positive Brudzinski's sign
   —positive Kernig's sign
   —drowsiness
   —vomiting

## Nursing Diagnosis
Altered Tissue Perfusion: Cerebral: Decreased Physiologic-Behavioral Responsiveness related to increased ICP.
*Desired outcome:* No signs or symptoms of increased ICP will occur. If they do, they will be recognized and reported to a doctor immediately.

### Interventions and rationales
1. Notify the doctor of the following signs and symptoms:
• change in orientation or level of consciousness (perform neurologic checks at least every hour)
• bradycardia or elevated blood pressure (check vital signs every hour)
• widening pulse pressure
• change in size, shape, equality, and reaction of pupils.
*Rationale:* These are signs of increasing ICP.
2. Notify the doctor immediately if you detect:
• sudden loss of consciousness
• a unilateral fixed, dilated pupil or bilateral pupillary changes
• sudden *pronounced* changes in vital signs (bradycardia, widening pulse pressure)
• sudden onset of gross neurologic deficit, such as hemiparesis, hemiplegia, facial paralysis, slurred speech, aphasia, or abnormal posturing in coma (see page 16).
*Rationale:* These can be ominous signs of brain stem compression or herniation requiring immediate treatment.
3. Limit fluids if not contraindicated.
*Rationale:* Fluid limitation decreases cerebral edema.

## Nursing Diagnosis
Potential for Injury: Trauma related to decreased awareness.
*Desired outcome:* Patient safety will be maintained.

### Interventions and rationales

1. Keep the side rails up at all times.
*Rationale:* The patient may become delirious and roll off the bed.
2. Use soft restraints if indicated.
*Rationale:* These help prevent serious injury if the patient is combative or disoriented.
3. Remain with the patient if he is very restless or delirious.
*Rationale:* A patient with altered perception may become frightened.

## Nursing Diagnosis

Impaired Skin Integrity related to immobility.
*Desired outcome:* No signs or symptoms of skin breakdown (pain, redness, blistering, necrosis, or tissue thinning) will occur.

### Interventions and rationales

1. Change the patient's position at least every 2 hours if he cannot do so himself. (He may benefit from an alternating-pressure mattress.)
*Rationale:* This relieves pressure over bony prominences, thereby helping to prevent skin breakdown.
2. Keep the patient's skin dry.
*Rationale:* Moisture encourages bacterial growth.
3. Massage around bony prominences.
*Rationale:* This increases circulation to the affected area.
4. Pad bony prominences if the patient is not on an alternating-pressure surface.
*Rationale:* This helps to distribute pressure and protect skin around bony prominences.
5. Inspect the skin for breakdown every 8 hours.
*Rationale:* Early detection of skin breakdown improves the chance of successful treatment.

## Nursing Diagnosis

Ineffective Breathing Pattern and Impaired Gas Exchange related to compression of brainstem from cerebral edema.
*Desired outcome:* Normal breathing pattern and ABG levels will be restored or maintained.

### Interventions and rationales

1. Monitor the patient's respiratory rate, pattern, and quality.
*Rationale:* Increased ICP can result in brain stem compression, affecting respirations.

2. Monitor ABG levels. Normal levels are $PaO_2$ from 80 to 100 mm Hg, $PaCO_2$ from 35 to 45 mm Hg, and pH from 7.35 to 7.45.
*Rationale:* ABG levels reflect the degree of ventilation.
3. Change the patient's position every 2 hours.
*Rationale:* This helps prevent additional respiratory complications, such as pooling of secretions and atelectasis.
4. Auscultate breath sounds every 2 hours and suction as needed.
*Rationale:* Coarse crackles or rhonchi indicate the need for suctioning or other attempts to mobilize secretions. (*Note:* Suctioning may be contraindicated with increased ICP.)

## Nursing Diagnosis
Impaired Physical Mobility related to decreased level of consciousness.
*Desired outcome:* No signs or symptoms of contracture will occur.

### Interventions and rationales
1. Maintain correct body alignment.
*Rationale:* This keeps extremities in a functional position and prevents hip contracture.
2. Provide range-of-motion exercises to all extremities every 8 hours.
*Rationale:* This helps keep the joints flexible.
3. Splint any paralyzed extremity.
*Rationale:* This helps maintain a functional limb position and prevents contracture.

## Medical Diagnosis
**Lumbar puncture** typically reveals elevated CSF pressure and protein content and depressed glucose levels. CSF culture and sensitivity tests usually reveal the causative organism.

**Chest X-ray** may reveal other areas of infection.

### Medical treatment
• specific antibiotic therapy to treat the causative organism
• sedatives to relieve restlessness
• mannitol to decrease cerebral edema
• analgesics to relieve pain
• antipyretics to reduce fever
• hypothermia, if indicated, for pyrexia (see page 92)
• isolation (depending on the causative organism)
• maintaining nutritional requirements and fluid and electrolyte balances

| FAMILY COPING | MENINGITIS |
|---|---|

*Whenever possible, actively involve the patient and family or significant other in discussing:*

• how the disease causes irritation of the membranes covering the brain and spinal cord
• diagnostic tests—the purpose, procedure, and how to obtain the results
• signs and symptoms that require immediate attention, including headaches, visual problems, and seizures
• the importance of seizure precautions.

## ☐ Migraine

Migraines are unilateral, throbbing, recurrent headaches commonly preceded by an aura. They are thought to result from vasoconstriction followed by vasodilation of cerebral blood vessels.

### Assessment

#### Frequently encountered subjective data

• severe, throbbing headache (unilateral or rarely bilateral)
• visual disturbances, such as the appearance of colored lights, light spots, wavy lines, blurred images, hemianopia (defective vision or blindness in half of the visual field), and photophobia
• nausea
• numbness in the hands and circumoral area
• hemiparesis (weakness on one side of the body)
• vertigo
• pain in the face and neck

#### Frequently encountered objective data

• vomiting
• diaphoresis
• pallor
• prostration
• red eyes, lacrimation

### Nursing Diagnosis:

Altered Comfort: Pain related to headache from vascular or allergic etiology.
*Desired outcome:* The patient verbalizes diminished or controlled pain.

## Interventions and rationales

1. Provide a quiet environment.
*Rationale:* Noise and activity can increase blood pressure and exacerbate headache pain.
2. Provide a darkened environment.
*Rationale:* This helps relieve photophobia and reduce squinting (which can cause an additional muscle tension headache).
3. Take vital signs every 30 minutes until the patient is stable.
*Rationale:* Blood pressure may be unstable, and medications and sedatives may affect vital signs.
4. Apply a cool, wet washcloth to the patient's forehead.
*Rationale:* This relieves flushing and surface vasodilation.
5. Have patient reduce tension by verbalizing his feelings.
*Rationale:* Verbalization of anger and other feelings toward illness can help relieve stress. Visitors can be a source of tension and may have to be limited.
6. Try therapeutic touch or other methods of pain control (such as biofeedback and visualization).
*Rationale:* These methods can help reduce the patient's anxiety level, which may diminish the pain.
7. Refer the patient to a pain control clinic if he has chronic migraine headaches.
*Rationale:* Long-term management provides the patient with a sense of self-control.

## Nursing Diagnosis

Knowledge Deficit related to the cause and management of migraine headache.
*Desired outcome:* The patient verbalizes an understanding of the causes of migraine headache and his treatment regimen.

### Interventions and rationales

1. Discuss with the patient events that precipitate his migraine.
*Rationale:* Avoiding precipitating factors can help prevent migraine attacks. (Some headaches follow ingestion of certain foods, such as wine, cheese, and chocolate.)
2. Discuss the migraine's cause and its relationship to headache onset.
*Rationale:* This helps dispel any misconceptions the patient may have about the disorder.

## Medical Diagnosis

**EEG** identifies the site of abnormal brain activity.

**Brain scan** can rule out a brain lesion.

**CT scan** rules out hemorrhage or a brain lesion.

**Lumbar puncture** rules out increased ICP and infection.

### Medical treatment
• ergotamine tartrate (given after onset of aura)
• aspirin or acetaminophen to relieve pain (given before narcotics or other medical treatments)
• narcotics to relieve pain unresponsive to other treatments
• propranolol to help reduce the frequency of headaches
• sedatives to promote rest (given as needed)
• methysergide to prevent or reduce the frequency of headaches (although serious adverse reactions may occur)
• antiemetics to control nausea (given as needed)

---

**FAMILY COPING** | **MIGRAINE**

*Whenever possible, actively involve the patient and family or significant other in discussing:*

• the specific type of headache that the doctor believes the patient is experiencing
• medications—actions, side effects, and administration
• the importance of avoiding bright lighting, bending, coughing, or any activity that increases intracranial pressure during a migraine
• precipitating factors and how to avoid them
• diagnostic tests—the purpose, procedure, and how to obtain the results.

## ☐ Multiple Sclerosis
Multiple sclerosis (MS) is a disorder characterized by progressive demyelination (destruction of the myelin sheath that covers and insulates nerves) of the brain and spinal cord white matter. MS causes varied signs and symptoms, depending on which CNS sections undergo demyelination. The prognosis also is variable. MS may progress rapidly, disabling the patient or causing death within months of the onset. However, about 70% of patients have prolonged remissions and lead active, productive lives.

### Assessment

#### Frequently encountered subjective data
• impaired visual acuity (diplopia)
• unilateral vision loss
• weakness and fatigability
• incontinence or retention of urine or feces

#### Frequently encountered objective data
• nystagmus (rapid eye movement toward and away from midline)
• motor or sensory disturbances, ataxia (lack of coordination), and paresthesia

- intention tremors
- spastic paralysis
- mood swings
- slurred speech
- hyperexcitability
- inappropriate affect

## Nursing Diagnosis
Self-Care Deficit (specify dressing, toileting, feeding, and so forth) related to weakness/spastic paralysis.
*Desired outcome:* The patient will assist with self-care within his physical limitations.

### Interventions and rationales
1. Assess the patient's ability to feed himself, perform personal hygiene, ambulate, and dress.
*Rationale:* This helps to establish a plan for assistance and to determine the need for assistive devices (see Section 4).
2. Teach the patient how to use assistive devices, and begin to discuss a discharge plan.
*Rationale:* Patients are anxious about adjusting to their home environment with additional handicaps. Discuss the patient's fears, and center your teaching on techniques and equipment that will be used after discharge as well as throughout his hospital stay.

## Nursing Diagnosis
Impaired Physical Mobility related to weakness and spasticity of extremities.
*Desired outcome:* Optimum mobility will be maintained. No signs or symptoms of contractures (joint pain, stiffness, or limited range of motion) will be present.

### Interventions and rationales
1. Provide range-of-motion exercises to all extremities every 8 hours.
*Rationale:* This stretches joint muscles, maintaining flexibility, and helps prevent or reduce muscle atrophy.
2. Have the patient do muscle-stretching exercises.
*Rationale:* Stretching reduces muscle spasticity.
3. Encourage ambulation.
*Rationale:* Ambulation prevents or reduces hazards of immobility.
4. Apply braces and splints if the patient has spasticity.
*Rationale:* These measures help prevent wrist contractures and footdrop.
5. Maintain proper body alignment while the patient is immobile.
*Rationale:* This keeps muscles and joints in a functional position.

## Nursing Diagnosis
Potential for Injury: Trauma related to altered mobility and sensory loss.
*Desired outcome:* No injuries will occur.

### Interventions and rationales
1. Teach the patient how to use assistive devices, such as walkers, canes, and braces.
*Rationale:* These devices can help the patient to avoid injury and encourage self-care.
2. Maintain an uncluttered environment, keeping frequently used articles within the patient's reach.
*Rationale:* This helps prevent injury to a visually impaired patient.
3. Avoid temperature extremes when bathing the patient or applying heat.
*Rationale:* This helps prevent burns if the patient has sensory loss.

## Nursing Diagnosis
Ineffective Airway Clearance related to dysphagia secondary to neuromuscular dysfunction.
*Desired outcome:* No signs or symptoms of choking (coughing, gasping, or inability to talk) will occur.

### Interventions and rationales
1. Keep suction equipment readily available.
*Rationale:* This may help reassure the patient if he is anxious.
2. Provide a suitable diet of soft, solid foods.
*Rationale:* These foods are more easily tolerated if the patient fears choking.

## Nursing Diagnosis
Impaired Gas Exchange related to immobility.
*Desired outcome:* No signs or symptoms of atelectasis or impaired gas exchange will occur.

### Interventions and rationales
1. Auscultate breath sounds every 2 hours in the acute patient.
*Rationale:* Observe the patient for crackles and rhonchi or diminished breath sounds that indicate lung congestion or consolidation.
2. Change the patient's position at least every 2 hours if the patient cannot do so himself.
*Rationale:* This mobilizes secretions and aerates lung sections compromised by positioning.
3. Encourage coughing and deep breathing.
*Rationale:* This helps mobilize secretions to be expelled.

4. Perform nasotracheal suctioning if lung sounds become congested.
*Rationale:* A clear airway leads to better gas exchange.

## Nursing Diagnosis
Impaired Skin Integrity related to immobility.
*Desired outcome:* No signs or symptoms of breakdown (pain, redness, blistering, necrosis, petechiae, or tissue thinness) will occur.

### Interventions and rationales
1. Examine the patient's skin for reddened areas once every 8 hours. Ask the patient about any pain or skin discomfort.
*Rationale:* Redness is the first sign of skin inflammation or breakdown.
2. Keep the patient's skin dry.
*Rationale:* Moisture encourages bacterial growth.
3. Massage around bony prominences.
*Rationale:* This increases circulation to areas of potential skin breakdown.
4. Place the patient on a flotation or alternating-pressure mattress or on a turning frame. Change his position at least every 2 hours.
*Rationale:* This helps alternate weight distribution and keeps pressure off bony prominences for prolonged periods.
5. Encourage adequate fluid intake if not contraindicated.
*Rationale:* This keeps the skin hydrated and thus discourages breakdown.

## Nursing Diagnosis
Urinary Retention related to abnormal sphincter control.
*Desired outcome:* No signs or symptoms of urinary tract infection (increased temperature, pain on urination, grossly bloody urine, or cloudy urine with sediment) will occur. No signs or symptoms of urinary retention (distended bladder on palpation, pain, and leaking or dribbling urine) will occur. Skin will remain dry.

### Interventions and rationales
1. Monitor fluid intake and output, noting elimination times.
*Rationale:* With normal intake, an interval longer than 4 to 6 hours between voidings could indicate retention and neuromuscular bladder complications.
2. Examine the patient's urine for gross blood, abnormal odor, cloudiness, and sediment.
*Rationale:* These are signs of urinary tract infection.
3. Request urinary catheterization if the patient is incontinent.

*Rationale:* This helps protect the skin and permits accurate intake and output measurement.

4. Teach intermittent catheterization if the patient or his family can master this task.

*Rationale:* Intermittent catheterization is preferred to indwelling (Foley) catheters, which have a higher rate of infection.

## Nursing Diagnosis
Knowledge Deficit related to etiology and prognosis of MS.
*Desired outcome:* The patient will verbalize an understanding of the signs and symptoms of his illness and its probable effects on activities of daily living and occupational skills.

### Interventions and rationales
1. Explore the patient's feelings about the illness.
*Rationale:* This helps alert the nurse to any misconceptions the patient may have.

2. Explain the probable disease progression (periods of exacerbation and remission) to the patient.
*Rationale:* Knowing that remission may last for months or, in some cases, years offers encouragement.

3. Encourage the patient to avoid physical and emotional stress whenever possible.
*Rationale:* Stress may exacerbate symptoms.

4. Explain to the patient that mood swings are an expected part of this illness.
*Rationale:* This helps allay anxieties the patient and his family may have concerning the patient's mental status.

5. Promote self-care within the patient's limitations.
*Rationale:* Self-care enhances self-esteem and discourages feelings of dependence.

## Medical Diagnosis
Multiple episodes of transient neurologic impairments and exacerbations and remissions are common MS signs and symptoms.

**Lumbar puncture** may show an elevated gamma globulin level with a normal or mildly elevated CSF protein level and an elevated CSF white blood cell count.

**CT scan** helps rule out spinal cord compression, a foramen magnum tumor, multiple small strokes, and syphilis or other infections.

**EEG** reveals abnormalities in about 30% of patients.

### Medical treatment
• adrenocorticotropic hormone (ACTH), prednisone, or dexamethasone to reduce associated edema of the myelin sheath
• chlordiazepoxide or diazepam to mitigate mood swings

| FAMILY COPING | MULTIPLE SCLEROSIS |
|---|---|

*Whenever possible, actively involve the patient and family or significant other in discussing:*

• the effects of demyelination on sensory and motor functions and factors that exacerbate the illness
• diagnostic tests—the purpose, procedure, and how to obtain the results
• medications—actions, side effects, and administration
• the importance of a balanced rest-activity cycle
• methods of conserving energy, such as sitting down for tasks, using electrical or automatic equipment, shopping at home, and wearing clothing that is easily put on and removed
• dietary changes using semisolid foods, if dysphagia is a problem
• routine bladder and bowel regimen and self-catheterization technique if ordered
• home safety measures
• local sources of additional help, such as home health care.

# ☐ Myasthenia Gravis

Myasthenia gravis is characterized by a failure in the transmission of nerve impulses at the neuromuscular junction that results in progressive, generalized weakness. Such impairment may be an autoimmune response, ineffective acetylcholine release, or inadequate muscle response to ACTH. Myasthenia gravis usually affects the muscles innervated by the cranial nerves (eyes, face, neck, and throat), but it can affect any muscle group. It has no known cure. When the disease involves the respiratory system, it may be life-threatening. Patients can lead relatively normal lives, except during periods of exacerbation.

## Assessment

### Frequently encountered subjective data
• muscle weakness and fatigue of voluntary muscles with exercise
• diplopia
• dysphagia and difficulty chewing
• difficulty breathing
• fear of choking

### Frequently encountered objective data
• muscle weakness or paralysis
• ptosis (drooping of the eyelids)
• expressionless face
• nasal vocal tones
• frequent choking episodes
• apparent respiratory muscle weakness

## Nursing Diagnosis

Self-Care Deficit (specify feeding, hygiene, dressing, ambulation, or toileting) related to generalized muscle weakness and fatigue. *Desired outcome:* The patient will assist with self-care to the extent of his capabilities.

### Interventions and rationales

1. Assess the patient's ability to:
- feed himself and drink liquids
- groom and dress himself
- perform personal hygiene
- ambulate
- transfer from the bed to a chair and back.

*Rationale:* This will help in developing a functional nursing care plan by specifying necessary physical assistance or assistive devices.

2. Arrange the patient's environment to provide easy access to frequently used items (depending on his degree of physical impairment).
*Rationale:* This helps provide for patient safety.

3. Plan the patient's activities in the morning or after short naps whenever possible.
*Rationale:* Energy peaks and muscle function is best during these times.

## Nursing Diagnosis

Impaired Verbal Communicaton related to hoarseness and inaudible speech secondary to weakness of vocal cords.
*Desired outcome:* An alternate method of communication will be established and used as needed.

### Interventions and rationales

1. Assess the patient's verbal abilities.
*Rationale:* This establishes a baseline for the nursing care plan.

2. Provide alternate methods of communication (such as picture cards, body signals, and special touch-sensitive call bells) based on the patient's needs.
*Rationale:* This decreases the patient's fear and frustration concerning his ability to communicate needs.

## Nursing Diagnosis

Potential Ineffective Breathing Pattern related to weakness of respiratory muscles.
*Desired outcome:* An effective breathing pattern will be maintained; the airway will be kept patent.

### Interventions and rationales

1. Keep suction, oxygen, and intubation equipment readily available.

*Rationale:* In many cases, stress may precipitate a myasthenic crisis, as can an overdose of anticholinergic drugs.

2. Monitor the patient for respiratory depression, indicated by a sudden exacerbation of muscle weakness resulting in dyspnea.

*Rationale:* Myasthenic crisis (acute disease exacerbation resulting in severely impaired respiratory effort from muscle weakness) is an emergency that requires the use of airway adjuncts and mechanical ventilation (see page 115). Know where to find emergency respiratory equipment on your unit.

3. Closely monitor the patient for respiratory difficulty 1 hour after each anticholinesterase dose.

*Rationale:* Cholinergic crisis may occur 1 hour after administering anticholinesterase drugs.

## Medical Diagnosis

Diagnosis comes primarily from clinical assessments based on characteristic fatigability seen in this disorder.

**Neostigmine methylsulfate (Prostigmin) test,** administered subcutaneously, produces relief of symptoms in 10 to 15 minutes and increased muscle strength in 30 minutes.

**Edrophonium chloride (Tensilon) test,** given intravenously, relieves symptoms in 30 seconds.

**Electromyography** determines the extent of muscle fatigability.

**Laboratory tests,** such as thyroxine and thyroid-stimulating hormone levels, are ordered to rule out thyroid disease.

### Medical treatment

• anticholinesterase drugs, such as ambenonium chloride (Mytelase), to inhibit acetylcholinesterase at the neuromuscular junction
• edrophonium chloride
• neostigmine methylsulfate
• pyridostigmine bromide (Mestinon)
• radiotherapy to decrease the size of the thymus gland, or surgery to remove it
• corticosteroid therapy to decrease the autoimmune response

---

**FAMILY COPING**   **MYASTHENIA GRAVIS**

---

*Whenever possible, actively involve the patient and family or significant other in discussing:*

• how the disease impairs transmission of nerve impulses, causing weakness and fatigue
• signs and symptoms requiring immediate attention, including difficulty swallowing, inability to cough, increased salivation, twitching around the eyes and mouth, nausea and vomiting, palpitations, muscle spasms, cold moist skin, confusion, seizures, and syncope

- diagnostic tests—the purpose, procedure, and how to obtain the results
- medications—actions, side effects, and the coordination of drug action with drug administration to take advantage of peak muscle strength
- dietary supplements to help compensate for muscle weakness
- factors that increase infection risk
- local sources of additional help, such as home health care.

# ☐ Parkinson's Disease

Parkinson's disease is a slow, progressively degenerative CNS disease that produces involuntary tremors, bradykinesia (slow movement), and muscle rigidity. Signs and symptoms of this disorder appear related to the loss of dopamine's inhibitory effect on the brain's caudate nucleus and putamen. Parkinson's disease progresses for an average of about 10 years, at which time death usually occurs from pneumonia or other complications.

## Assessment

### Frequently encountered subjective data
- muscle rigidity or tremors
- dysphagia
- fatigue

### Frequently encountered objective data
- nonintentional tremors that increase when the limb is at rest and cease with voluntary movement
- fixed facial expression with unblinking stare
- slowed body movements
- shuffling gait with a tendency to accelerate and fall forward
- drooling

## Nursing Diagnosis

Impaired Physical Mobility related to rigidity and tremors.
*Desired outcome:* Optimum mobility will be maintained.

### Interventions and rationales
1. Gather baseline data on the patient's gait, muscular rigidity, tremors, and voluntary movements.
*Rationale:* This helps determine the patient's capacity for self-care.
2. Encourage the patient to maintain activities of daily living.
*Rationale:* This discourages dependence and enhances self-esteem.
3. Refer the patient to a physical therapist.
*Rationale:* The patient requires a daily exercise regimen with range-of-motion exercises to remain flexible.

## Nursing Diagnosis

Altered Nutrition: Less than Body Requirements: Decreased Intake related to chewing/swallowing difficulties and inability to feed or drink fluids without help.

*Desired outcome:* Optimum nutrition will be maintained; no undesired weight loss will occur.

### Interventions and rationales

1. Assess the patient's ability to chew and swallow food.
*Rationale:* This helps you to plan his diet appropriately; soft, solid foods are best.
2. Assess the ability of the patient to drink fluids and feed himself.
*Rationale:* This helps determine if the patient needs assistance with feeding or if he should receive smaller, more frequent meals, with adequate time allowed for finishing them.
3. Help the patient select an appropriate diet.
*Rationale:* The patient needs adequate fiber to prevent constipation and adequate fluid intake.

## Nursing Diagnosis

Self-Care Deficit (specify dressing, toileting, feeding, and so forth) related to muscle rigidity and tremors.

*Desired outcome:* The patient will perform hygiene, toileting, and dressing activities within the scope of his capabilities.

### Interventions and rationales

1. Assess the patient's ability to eat, bathe, dress, and perform toileting functions (including ambulation to the bathroom or use of a bedside commode or bedpan).
*Rationale:* This allows you to develop a plan to meet the patient's physical assistance needs or to provide assistive devices.
2. Implement a plan designed for the patient to follow one step at a time. Allow rest periods between activities.
*Rationale:* Patients fatigue quite easily. A routine schedule that provides rest periods makes tasks easier on the patient.

## Nursing Diagnosis

Dysfunction Grieving: Depression related to physical limitations and body image changes.

*Desired outcome:* The patient will progress normally through the grieving process related to physical loss. He will eventually exhibit no signs or symptoms of clinical depression.

### Interventions and rationales

1. Assess the patient's coping status and potential for suicide.
*Rationale:* The patient already may have attempted or threatened suicide since the onset of the disease, which may necessitate close observation.

2. Encourage the patient to express his feelings.
*Rationale:* Parkinson's disease can lead to feelings of hopelessness. If the patient expresses such feelings, appropriate strategies can be developed based on his strengths.
3. Involve the patient in activities with others, especially those with similar disorders. Select activities that foster self-esteem.
*Rationale:* This helps the patient focus on activities outside of himself and deal with his capabilities.
4. Teach the patient about his drug regimen if he's receiving antidepressants.
*Rationale:* Certain antidepressants necessitate dietary restrictions (check with the pharmacist). The patient should understand the adverse reactions, length of treatment, and length of time associated with the onset of symptom relief.
5. Teach the patient constructive problem-solving techniques, and discuss alternatives to situations that the patient perceives as hopeless.
*Rationale:* Depression may alter the patient's perception of reality, so he may benefit from discussing options and alternatives to stressors with an objective listener.

## Medical Diagnosis
Parkinson's disease is diagnosed clinically, based on physical findings, such as resting tremors and cogwheel rigidity (jerks with alternating periods of rest during passive limb movement).

**EEG** may reveal abnormal findings.

### Medical treatment
• Sinemet (a mixture of levodopa and carbidopa)
• anticholinergics
• antihistamines
• antidepressants
• bromocriptine (may produce clinical improvement when dopamine loses its effectiveness)
• physical therapy

| FAMILY COPING | PARKINSON'S DISEASE |
| --- | --- |

*Whenever possible, actively involve the patient and family or significant other in discussing:*

• the progressive decline associated with the disease and the need to establish a plan for care during the later stages
• diagnostic tests—the purpose, procedure, and how to obtain the results
• dietary restrictions
• an exercise program to maintain range of motion or flexibility suited to the patient's stage of illness
• assistive devices and techniques for dressing, walking, and other activities of daily living

• measures for preventing orthostatic hypotension
• home safety measures, such as removing throw rugs and unstable furniture
• signs and symptoms of clinical depression and when to seek professional help
• local sources of additional help, such as home health care and support groups.

## ☐ Tumor, Cerebral

Whether benign or malignant, a brain tumor is dangerous because its continued growth results in local tissue irritation and increased ICP. Malignant brain tumors can be classified as gliomas or schwannomas, depending on the nervous tissue of origin, or as metastatic tumors. Most are supratentorial (above the covering of the cerebellum). Patients with brain tumors have the same signs and symptoms as patients with other space-occupying lesions in the brain. As they increase in size, they can cause a shift in midline structures and eventual herniation of brain tissue.

### Assessment
#### Frequently encountered subjective data
(depending on the affected area of the brain)
• headache
• weakness
• motor and sensory deficits
• visual disturbances
• nausea

#### Frequently encountered objective data
• confusion
• seizures
• papilledema
• abnormal pupillary response
• motor and sensory deficits
• increased ICP
• decreased level of consciousness
• personality changes or aberrant behavior
• vomiting

### Nursing Diagnosis
Altered Tissue Perfusion: Cerebral: Decreased Physiologic-Behavioral Responsiveness related to increased ICP.
*Desired outcome:* No signs or symptoms of increased ICP will occur. If they do occur, they will be recognized and reported immediately.

## HERNIATION: TWO TYPES

In brain herniation, increased ICP forces brain tissue through the tentorial notch (uncal herniation) or the foramen magnum (brain stem herniation).

### Uncal herniation

As the illustration below shows, the dura flares out from the posterior part of the falx cerebri, forming the tentorium cerebelli. The cerebral hemispheres lie above the tentorium (supratentorial); the cerebellum and brain stem lie below the tentorium (infratentorial).

Any abnormal mass that takes up intracranial space is called a *space-occupying lesion*. Examples include tumors, aneurysms, hematomas, and abscesses. By taking up space, they can increase intracranial pressure (ICP). Or, in some cases, they can irritate and compress adjacent brain tissue, causing brain damage and dysfunction without an overall increase in ICP. In uncal herniation, a supratentorial space-occupying lesion causes part of the temporal lobe called the uncus to be forced through the tentorial notch.

Pressure on this brain tissue produces the following signs and symptoms:
• a unilateral, dilated pupil that turns outward

• decreased level of consciousness, with rapid deterioration to coma
• impaired motor function (initially ipsilateral, then bilateral).

As the patient's condition deteriorates:
• The doll's eye reflex becomes difficult to elicit, then disappears.
• Cheyne-Stokes breathing progresses to central neurogenic hyperventilation.
• Dilated pupils become fixed at midpoint.
• He has purposeful responses to noxious stimulus initially, but eventually assumes decerebrate posturing. (Rigidity may also be present.)

### Brain stem herniation

Signs and symptoms that the brain stem has herniated through the foramen magnum include:
• coma
• fixed, dilated pupils
• absent doll's eye reflex
• flaccid response to noxious stimulus
• bilateral Babinski's reflexes (see page 12)
• widely varying pulse rate
• gradual blood pressure drop.

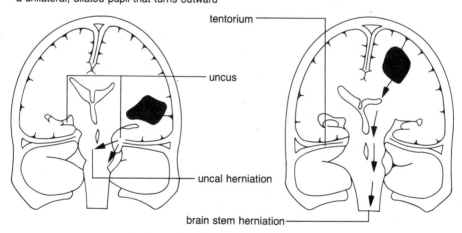

tentorium

uncus

uncal herniation

brain stem herniation

### Interventions and rationales

1. Monitor the patient for:
• change in level of consciousness or orientation (perform neurologic checks at least every hour)
• bradycardia (take vital signs at least every hour)
• widening pulse pressure
• size, shape, equality, and reaction of pupils.
*Rationale:* These signs and symptoms can warn of increased ICP.
2. Notify the doctor immediately if you detect:
• unilateral, fixed, dilated pupil
• sudden loss of consciousness
• sudden pronounced changes in vital signs (for example, bradycardia or increased blood pressure)
• sudden onset of gross neurologic deficit, such as hemiparesis, hemiplegia, facial paralysis, slurred speech, aphasia, or abnormal posturing in coma.
*Rationale:* These may be ominous signs of brain stem compression or herniation requiring immediate treatment by a neurosurgeon.
3. Limit fluids if not contraindicated.
*Rationale:* This decreases cerebral edema.

## Nursing Diagnosis

Potential for Injury: Trauma related to loss of awareness and loss of motor control secondary to seizures.
*Desired outcome:* The patient's seizures will be controlled medically. If seizures occur, they will be treated promptly and patient safety will be maintained.

### Interventions and rationales

Take the following seizure precautions:
• Keep a soft oral airway or rolled washcloth taped to the headboard.
• Have emergency drugs, such as I.V. diazepam, phenytoin, and phenobarbital, readily accessible.
• Provide a quiet atmosphere.
• Decrease lighting in the patient's room.
• Avoid nonessential procedures.
• Pad bed rails; keep them up when the patient is in bed.
• Take no oral temperatures using a glass thermometer.
• Do not allow unsupervised smoking.
*Rationale:* These measures provide for the patient's safety and decrease activity that may stimulate seizures.

## Nursing Diagnosis

Alterations in Comfort related to headache pain secondary to space-occupying lesion.

*Desired outcome:* The patient will state that the headache pain has been managed or diminished.

### Interventions and rationales

1. Administer analgesic medications as needed.
*Rationale:* The patient will probably require medication to diminish pain.
2. Provide bed rest and a quiet environment. Avoid quick or jarring movements.
*Rationale:* Jarring causes movement of the mass and increased pain.
3. Decrease lighting in the patient's room.
*Rationale:* Even if the patient isn't photophobic, lighting may make him squint excessively, resulting in an additional muscle tension headache.

## Medical Diagnosis

**CT scan** will reveal a space-occupying lesion or mass.

**MRI** also may reveal a space-occupying lesion or mass, but in more detail than a CT scan.

**Skull X-rays** can reveal a mass or shift in the pineal body.

**Arteriography** shows displacement of major vessels or outlines of the neoplasm.

**Brain scan** shows the presence of a space-occupying lesion.

### Medical treatment
• surgical management by excision
• irradiation
• chemotherapy
• osmotic diuretics to decrease cerebral edema
• corticosteroids
• anticonvulsants
• analgesics

| FAMILY COPING | CEREBRAL TUMOR |
| --- | --- |

*Whenever possible, actively involve the patient and family or significant other in discussing:*

• increased intracranial pressure and how it causes subtle behavioral changes, such as restlessness, confusion, and disorientation
• signs and symptoms requiring immediate attention, such as headache, visual changes, lethargy, or syncope as well as numbness, paralysis, or weakness
• medications—actions, side effects, and administration
• diagnostic tests—the purpose, procedure, and how to obtain the results
• surgery, if indicated.

# 4 Special Equipment and Assistive Interventions

The following special equipment and assistive interventions are arranged in alphabetical order.

## ☐ Aphasia Board

### Purpose
To facilitate communication with patients who cannot speak.

### Description
A board or piece of paper with pictures of frequently used items, such as a water glass or a bedpan.

### Interventions
Approach the patient from his unaffected side with consideration for any visual problems. Have the patient point to the picture of what he needs. If he cannot point, develop a signal he can use as you point to various items. Aphasia boards are easy to make from magazine clippings if a commercial one is not available.

## ☐ Canes

### Purpose
To provide stability for patients with unsteady gait.

### Description
Besides the familiar wooden cane with a hook-shaped handle, there are several types of metal canes:
• standard hook top for patients needing slight assistance
• T-handle for patients with hand weakness
• quadripod cane with broad base used for patients with one-sided weakness who are unable to use walker.

### Interventions
To adjust a cane, find the correct height (handle should be level with the greater trochanter, allowing a 15-degree elbow flexion), then push in the metal buttons and slide to the appropriate length. Instruct the patient to hold the cane with his unaffected hand, distribute his weight away from the affected side, and achieve a reciprocal, balanced gait.

## ☐ CircOlectric (Circle) Bed

### Purpose
To turn severely burned, injured, or immobilized patients.

## Description

The CircOlectric is an anterior-posterior frame bed attached to a circular turning device. It provides for vertical as opposed to lateral turning of the patient and is operated electrically. The bed can be used on patients with cervical traction, since traction can be maintained throughout the vertical turning procedure.

## Interventions

This procedure is not to be performed without consulting the manufacturer's directions and your hospital procedure manual. If you have never operated the bed, obtain the assistance of your instructor or a nurse experienced in the procedure before you begin to prepare the patient. Before turning the patient, clear all tubing and traction weights. If the patient is on a respirator, use a bag-valve device (Ambu bag) while turning. Do not pause while turning (this can be disturbing to a patient); instead, turn the bed slowly, continually monitoring patient response. In patients with spinal cord injuries, extreme care must be taken to avoid severe hypotensive episodes associated with rapid changes in position.

*Note:* CircOlectric beds are contraindicated for unstable spine disorders because the feet bear much of the weight in turning.

With the patient in a supine position, follow these general directions:

• basic preparation
  —Center the patient's hips at the gatch.
  —Adjust the footboard to prevent the patient from sliding down during a transfer revolution.
  —Pad legs and knees with pillows.
  —Use a sponge face protector over the patient's face.
• frame application
  —Place the anterior frame over the patient.

### THE CIRCOLECTRIC BED

To ensure patient safety, as one nurse turns the bed, the other nurse watches and reassures the patient.

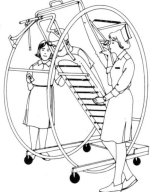

—Lock it in place with a stud and nut bolt.

—Apply a safety strap if the patient cannot control his arms.

• turning

—Tell the patient the direction you will be turning.

—Begin slow bed rotation, using a remote switch controller.

—Complete rotation until patient is parallel with the floor.

• posterior frame removal

—Remove the posterior stud nut from the frame head.

—Press the safety bar forward to disengage the posterior section.

—Raise the posterior section overhead and lock it into the circle frame with the safety bar.

## ☐ Cradle Boots

### Purpose
To prevent footdrop, external hip rotation, and skin breakdown.

### Description
Cradle boots consist of foam blocks with a superior slit and a cutout interior.

### Interventions
Open the superior slit and place the supine patient's aligned leg in the cutout area. Place the boot on the bottom leg only when the patient is lying on his side.

## ☐ Decubitus Ulcer Care

### Purpose
To promote healing of tissue injured by ischemia caused by pressure.

### Description
Treatment of decubitus ulcers involves prevention of further tissue injury by alleviating pressure on the affected area, increasing circulation to the tissues, keeping the area clean and free of infection, and improving nutrition.

### Interventions
Intervention depends on the level of tissue damage. For specific treatments, assess the decubitus ulcer and use the chart at right as a guide for treatment.

## ☐ Eye Care

### Purpose
To prevent corneal injury in comatose patients or those with eyelid paralysis.

# UNDERSTANDING DECUBITUS ULCERS

| Description | Treatment | Nursing considerations |
|---|---|---|
| **Stage 1** Epidermal redness, no induration | • Increase circulation to reddened area by massaging around decubitus ulcer*. • Relieve pressure over site; avoid positioning on affected area. | • Turn at least every 2 hours. • Keep skin dry. |
| **Stage 2** Swelling, redness, induration, possible epidermal blistering | • Relieve pressure over site; avoid positioning on affected area. • Increase circulation to reddened area by massaging around decubitus ulcer*. • Prevent infection by keeping skin clean and dry. • Assess nutritional status. | • Turn every 2 hours. |
| **Stage 3** Necrosis of epidermis with exposure of underlying fat | • Relieve pressure over site; avoid positioning on affected area. • Increase circulation by massaging around affected area and applying medical stimulant, if ordered. • Prevent or treat existing infection with dressings and medications, as ordered. • Assess supplemental nutritional needs. | • Turn every 2 hours. • Order a diet high in protein and vitamin C, if appropriate. • Debride affected area. • Prepare patient for possible surgical intervention. |
| **Stage 4** Epidermal and fat necrosis to muscle layer | • Relieve pressure over site; do not position on affected area. • Increase circulation by massaging lightly around area. • Prevent or treat existing infection, with medications, as ordered. • Assess supplemental nutritional needs. | • Turn every 2 hours. • Order a diet high in protein and vitamin C, if appropriate. • Debride and apply topical antibiotics, with periodic dressing changes and irrigation as ordered. • Prepare patient for possible surgical intervention. |
| **Stage 5** Epidermal fat and muscle necrosis | • Relieve pressure over site; do not position on affected area. • Débride necrotic tissue with dressing changes and irrigation, as ordered. • Treat infection, as ordered. • Assess supplemental nutritional needs. | • Turn every 2 hours. • Order a diet high in protein and vitamin C, if appropriate. • Prepare patient for sugery (needed in most cases). |
| **Stage 6** Bone involvement | • Relieve pressure over site; do not position on affected area. • Remove necrotic tissue with dressings and irrigation, as ordered. • Treat infection, as ordered. • Assess supplemental nutritional needs. | • Consider special beds that reduce pressure over bony prominences†. • Order a diet high in protein and vitamin C, if appropriate. • Prepare patient for surgery. |
| **Stage 7** Osteomyelitis; severe bone penetration with possible fracture | • Remove necrotic tissue with frequent dressing changes and irrigation, as ordered. • Control infection with medications, as ordered. • Assess supplemental nutritional needs. | • Consider use of special bed to reduce pressure over bony prominences; do not position patient on affected area. • Encourage a diet high in protein, vitamin C, and calories, if appropriate. • Prepare patient for surgery. |

* Massage the surrounding area—not the decubitus ulcer itself. Massaging over an indurated area can cause further tissue damage and will not promote circulation but only result in further skin breakdown.
† Find out what equipment is preferred and what adjuncts to decubitus care are available in your hospital by consulting the patient's doctor and others, such as the physical therapist. Possibilities include flotation, CircOlectric, and Roto Rest beds as well as Stryker and Foster frames.
Adapted from Conway-Rutkowski, B.: *Carini and Owens' Neurological-Neurosurgical Nursing,* 8th ed. St. Louis: C.V. Mosby Co., 1982.

### Description
The procedure varies with doctor preference. The aim is to keep corneas moist and protected from injury.

### Interventions
Remove secretions and crusts from around the eyelid and lashes with saline solution–soaked pads. Work from the inner canthus to the outer eye area. Use a clean pad for each wipe. Never use the same pad on both eyes. Instill artificial tears or ointment if ordered. Cover one or both eyes with a pad secured with hypoallergenic tape.

## ☐ Feeding Devices

### Large-Handled Utensils

### Purpose
To facilitate grasping of utensil.

### Description
Large handles compensate for the patient's weakened grasp.

### Interventions
Allow the patient to experiment, using a plate guard.

### Long-Handled Utensils

### Purpose
To help patients with limited shoulder and elbow movement to lift food to the mouth.

### Description
These large-handled, jointed utensils can be adjusted to accommodate decreased range of motion in the arm.

### Interventions
Allow the patient to experiment with the device, moving food across the plate toward him. Use with a plate guard.

### Plate Guards

### Purpose
To help put food on utensils without pushing it off the plate.

### Description
This circular ring attaches to a plate and prevents spills. It is frequently used with other assistive feeding devices.

## ASSISTIVE FEEDING DEVICES

Various devices can help the patient with limited arm mobility, grasp, range of motion, or coordination to feed himself.

Before introducing your patient to an assistive feeding device, assess his ability to master it. Don't introduce a device he can't manage. If his condition is progressively disabling, encourage him to use the device only until his mastery of it falters.

Introduce the assistive device before mealtime, with the patient seated in a natural position. Explain its purpose, show the patient how to use it, and encourage him to practice using it.

After meals, wash the device thoroughly and store it in the patient's bedside stand so it doesn't get misplaced. Document the patient's progress and share breakthroughs with staff and family members to help reinforce the patient's independence. Devices you can use include the following:

• **Plate guards** help all patients who have difficulty feeding themselves. The guard blocks food from spilling off the plate, allowing it to be picked up with a fork or spoon. Attach the guard to the side of the plate opposite the hand the patient uses to feed himself. Guiding the patient's hand, show him how to push food against the guard to secure it on the utensil. Then have him try again with food of a different consistency. When the patient tires, feed him the rest of the meal. At subsequent meals, encourage the patient to feed himself for progressively longer periods until he can feed himself an entire meal.

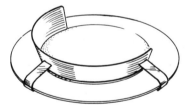

• **Swivel spoons** can help the patient with limited range of motion in his forearm. They can be used with universal cuffs.

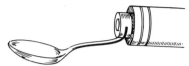

• **Universal cuffs** help the patient with flail hands or diminished grasp. The cuff contains a slot that holds a fork or spoon. Attach it to the hand the patient uses to feed himself. Then, place a fork or spoon in the cuff slot. If necessary, bend the utensil to facilitate feeding.

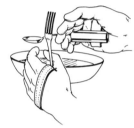

• **Long-handled utensils** can help the patient with limited range of motion in his elbow and shoulder.

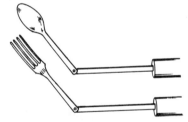

• **Utensils with built-up handles** can help the patient with diminished grasp. They are commercially available but can also be improvised by wrapping tape around the handle of a fork or spoon.

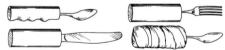

### Interventions

Attach the guard to the side of the plate opposite the hand that the patient uses to eat. Guide the patient's hand, showing him how to push food against the guard and onto the utensil.

## Swivel Spoons

### Purpose

To pick up food for patients with limited forearm movement.

### Description

The spoon has a large handle that can be grasped easily or used with a universal cuff. The bowl tips to facilitate emptying.

### Interventions

Assess the patient's ability to use the device. Determine if a universal cuff is needed (the spoon handle fits into the cuff).

## Universal Cuff

### Purpose

To help patients with diminished hand strength to hold utensils.

### Description

The cuff surrounds the hand and has a slot for utensils.

### Interventions

Place a utensil in the cuff slot, and fasten the cuff to the patient's hand. Bend the utensil if necessary. Allow the patient to practice using the cuff.

## ☐ Halo Traction

### Purpose

To immobilize cervical vertebrae after injury. This allows the patient to ambulate with skeletal traction (unlike skeletal tongs).

### Description

A metal halo ring is attached to a plastic vest with bar supports (see *Halo Device* at right).

### Interventions

Notify the doctor if the pins or vest becomes dislodged or misaligned or if the patient has a sudden motor or sensory loss. Cleanse the pin sites on the skull every 4 hours with hydrogen

## HALO DEVICE

Another form of skeletal immobilizer for patients with cervical injuries is the halo device.

For this, the doctor places an adjustable stainless steel hoop around the patient's head and secures it to his skull with two occipital and two temporal screws. Steel bars anchor this device to the patient's body cast or sheepskin-lined vest.

The halo allows your patient greater mobility, with minimal risk of disturbing his spinal alignment during position changes. He's usually permitted out of bed earlier than a patient with skull tongs because the alignment can be maintained more easily.

You'll probably care for your patient with a halo in a regular hospital bed. Place him on either side, as well as supine or prone. Do not elevate his head or legs. In the acute phase, you may wish to avoid the prone position. Not only does this position make respiratory assessment more difficult, but it may also disturb the patient whose face is inches away from the mattress.

Get assistance when changing your patient's position every 2 hours. Use a pull sheet. Lift but don't drag him to the side of the bed. Then roll him to the desired position; never turn or lift him by grabbing the halo.

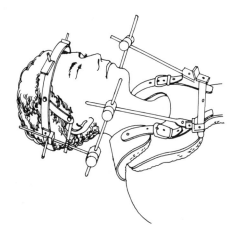

If a pin becomes detached from the halo, don't move the patient. Call the doctor. Stabilize the patient's head with your hands until the doctor arrives.

*Nursing tip:* Your patient in skull tongs or halo traction will be especially sensitive to any noise made by striking the metal since bone is an excellent sound conductor. Avoid letting anything hit these metal devices.

peroxide on cotton-tipped applicators. Apply povidone-iodine dressing if the sites are infected. Wash the patient's chest and back (after loosening Velcro vest straps) daily. Dry the area thoroughly, preferably with a hair dryer on the cool setting. Observe for reddened pressure areas.

# ☐ Hand Rolls

## Purpose

May prevent flexion contractures of the hand; frequently used on hemiplegic patients when splints are not available.

## Description

A rolled washcloth can be substituted and held in place with gauze.

### Interventions

Place the hand roll in the patient's hand between his thumb and forefinger, wrapping the fingers around the sides. Fasten the Velcro strap. Not everyone agrees that hand rolls can actually prevent flexion contractures, because they encourage flexion of the fingers.

## ☐ Hypothermia Blanket

### Purpose

Most often used to lower body temperature when antipyretics are not effective. The hypothermia blanket also can be used to raise body temperature.

### Description

The large metal control unit on a wheeled frame has front jacks for a thermistor probe, a skin probe (axillary), and an esophageal probe. It uses coolant (usually distilled water and 20% ethyl alcohol), which is pumped through the blanket. A reservoir cap is usually on top of the unit. See the manufacturer's directions.

### Interventions

Hypothermia blankets should be used cautiously in patients with impaired peripheral circulation; severe tissue damage may result. Cover the hypothermia blanket with a bath blanket to absorb condensation and place both under the patient. (Sometimes a second hypothermia blanket is used to cover the patient.) Follow the manufacturer's directions for operation in either the manual or automatic mode (automatic mode uses a rectal, skin, or esophageal probe and automatically adjusts temperature until a preset limit is obtained).

## ☐ Intracranial Pressure Monitoring

### Purpose

To directly monitor intracranial pressure via catheter-transducer or fiberoptic sensor systems.

### Description

There are three types of intracranial pressure (ICP) monitoring devices:

**Ventricular catheterization.** A silicon rubber catheter is inserted into the lateral ventricle through a twist drill hole. Although it is the most accurate type of ICP monitoring, it has the greatest risk of infection. The catheter is connected to a pressur-

## THREE TYPES OF I.C.P. MONITORING

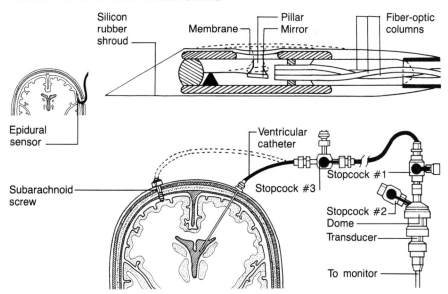

In **ventricular catheter monitoring,** which directly monitors intracranial pressure (ICP), the doctor inserts a small polyethylene or silicone rubber catheter into the lateral ventricle through a twist drill burr hole. Although this method measures ICP most accurately, it carries the greatest risk of infection. Placing the catheter may be difficult, especially if the ventricle is collapsed, swollen, or displaced. However, this is the only type of ICP monitoring that allows for evaluation of brain compliance and drainage of significant amounts of cerebrospinal fluid (CSF).

**Subarachnoid screw monitoring** involves the insertion of an ICP screw into the subarachnoid space through a twist drill burr hole in the front of the skull behind the hairline. Placing an ICP screw is easier than placing a ventricular catheter, especially if a computed tomography (CT) scan reveals shifting of the cerebrum or collapsed ventricles. This type of ICP monitoring also carries less risk of infection and parenchymal damage because

the screw doesn't penetrate the cerebrum.

In *both* ventricular catheter and subarachnoid screw monitoring (see illustration above), a fluid-filled line connects the catheter or screw to a domed transducer. Elevated ICP exerts pressure on the fluid in the line, depressing the transducer's diaphragm. The transducer then transmits pressure readings to a monitor for display. If desired, the readings can also be transmitted to a recorder for readout strips.

**Epidural sensor monitoring,** the least invasive method with the lowest incidence of infection, uses a fiber-optic sensor inserted into the epidural space through a burr hole (see illustration above). A cable connects the sensor to a monitor and, if desired, to a recorder. Unlike a ventricular catheter or subarachnoid screw, the sensor can't become occluded with blood or brain tissue. However, the accuracy of epidural monitoring is questionable because it doesn't measure ICP directly from a cranial space filled with CSF.

ized flush irrigation system and a monitoring device that uses a diaphragm to detect pressure and convert it to oscilloscopic waveforms (transducer).

**Subarachnoid screw.** A catheter is inserted into the subarachnoid space through a twist drill hole in the skull. Although the subarachnoid screw is easier to place and less dangerous than a ventricular catheter, it cannot drain off as much cerebrospinal fluid. The subarachnoid screw uses a pressurized flush system and transducer.

**Epidural sensor.** A fiberoptic sensor is inserted through a twist drill hole into the epidural space to measure ICP indirectly (pressure of dura against skull). Although the least accurate of these three monitors, it poses the least amount of risk to the patient.

### Interventions
Care of monitored patients includes the following:
• Perform neurologic checks at least every hour.
• Use all known methods of decreasing ICP:
  —Oxygenate before suctioning.
  —Elevate the head of the bed 30 degrees (check that the transducer is in the proper position).
  —Avoid neck flexion.
  —Have the patient avoid Valsalva's maneuver and straining.
  —Keep pressure lines patent (most doctors recommend not flushing unless absolutely necessary since this raises ICP).
  —Monitor wave patterns (normal ICP ranges from 5 to 15 mm Hg).
• Change dressings on the catheter site every 24 hours. Use occlusive dressings with povidone-iodine or other antifungal or antibacterial ointments. The major complication of these procedures is infection.
• Know how to operate equipment. Operating sophisticated equipment and performing procedures that pose a significant risk for the patient, such as ICP monitoring, require direct supervision by an experienced clinician. Neither nurses nor students should attempt to manage this area of patient care without previous training.

## ☐ Jackson-Pratt Drain

### Purpose
To drain the subdural space postoperatively.

### Description

The Jackson-Pratt drain is an oval, clear, pliable reservoir connected to a drain tube. The drain is activated by compressing the bulb to restore a vacuum once the contents have been emptied through a capped opening.

### Interventions

The drain is usually left in place 24 to 48 hours postoperatively. Empty and record output at least every 8 hours. Open the valve and drain contents from the bulb, using sterile procedure. Squeeze the bulb and close the valve to reestablish suction.

**JACKSON-PRATT SUCTION DRAIN**

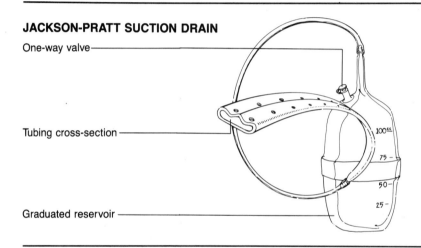

One-way valve

Tubing cross-section

Graduated reservoir

## ☐ Logrolling

### Purpose

To maintain spinal alignment while turning the patient.

### Description

A maneuver used to turn a reclining patient without flexing the spinal column.

### Interventions

The patient's bed should be made with a draw sheet. Three people are needed to turn the patient: One is positioned to hold his head in alignment while turning, one at the side of the bed turns the supine patient's trunk using a draw sheet, and the third turns the patient's legs to prevent twisting of the lower spine. Use foam wedges or pillows to position the patient in proper side alignment with a small pillow under his head.

## ☐ Positioning: Flat, Prone, and Side-Lying

### Purpose

To maintain proper body alignment in order to prevent such functional problems as hip rotation contracture.

### Description

In immobile patients, three basic positions relieve pressure on the skin over bony prominences. Repositioning allows for increased circulation to these areas and maintains skin integrity.

### Interventions

Follow the chart below. Change the immobile patient's position every 2 hours. Pad areas with wedges, pillows, or both.

**THREE COMMON POSITIONS**

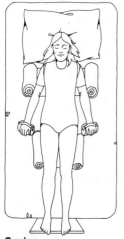

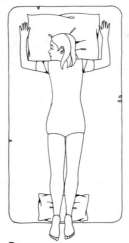

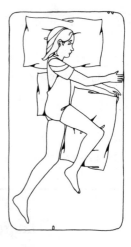

**Supine**
Place the patient on her back, with her face upward. Use shoulder, hand, and trochanter rolls and footboard to position and align the patient's extremities.

**Prone**
Place the patient on her stomach, with her face to the side.

**Lateral**
Place the patient on one side, with her head aligned with her spine and her body straight.

## ☐ Range-of-Motion Exercises, Passive

### Purpose

To prevent joint contractures in immobile patients.

### Description

Each joint should be taken through complete range of motion while the patient is supine. This includes adduction, abduction, flexion, extension, and rotation of neck (if not contraindicated), shoulders, elbow, wrist, fingers, arm, hip joint, leg, knee, ankle, and toes.

## Interventions

All range-of-motion exercises should be performed for immobile patients every 4 hours.

## RANGE-OF-MOTION EXERCISES

The purpose of passive (no patient participation) and active (patient participation) range-of-motion (ROM) exercises is to preserve joint mobility and prevent contractures in an immobile patient. During the procedure, each joint is taken through its normal pattern of movement. An easy way to remember the steps involved is to think of your own joints and how they normally move. Start with your patient's head and work toward his feet.

Before beginning range-of-motion exercises, you must check to see if any of them are contraindicated. For example, you certainly wouldn't move your patient's neck if a

fracture was suspected. Next, you must determine which exercises, if any, the patient is able to do himself (active ROM). If he is able to perform the exercises without assistance, you will need to teach him how to go about it. The illustrations below and on page 98 show normal range of joint movement.

If your patient is comatose or unable to move, you must do this for him to the extent that you are able (passive ROM). If the patient is conscious, do not force joints against painful resistance. Use the range-of-motion chart for reference, with the patient supine or turned side-to-side as needed.

**Shoulder**

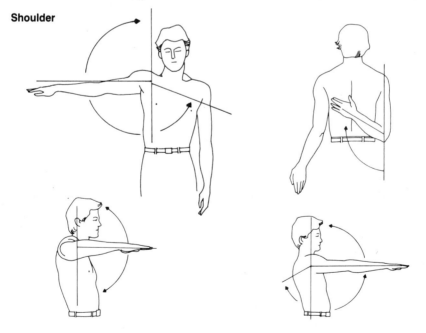

*(continued)*

## RANGE-OF-MOTION EXERCISES *(continued)*

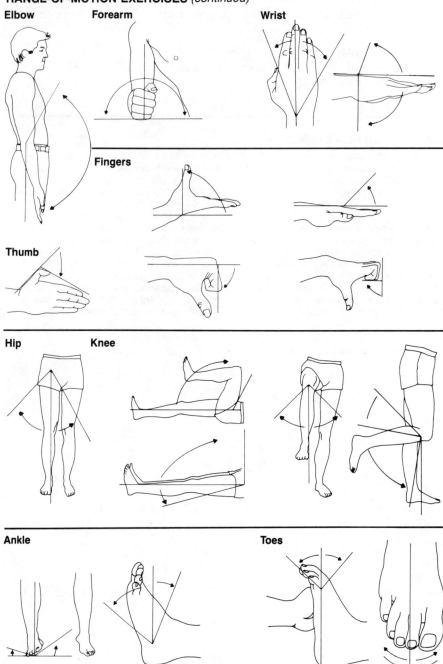

Elbow  Forearm  Wrist

Fingers

Thumb

Hip  Knee

Ankle  Toes

# ☐ Roto Rest Bed

### Purpose

To provide constant passive exercise and peristaltic stimulation. The bed shifts body weight to eliminate prolonged pressure on bony prominences.

### Description

The bed rotates 14 times per hour. It has a built-in fan for cooling the patient or reducing fever.

### Interventions

Use padded accessories to hold the patient in place and to prevent shearing forces. If the patient is an amputee, place sandbags in the appropriate area to balance the bed. Incontinent patients should be diapered because the numerous cushions are difficult to clean. The bed is radiolucent, so X-rays may be taken without moving the patient. Review the manufacturer's directions before operating bed.

**ROTO REST BED**

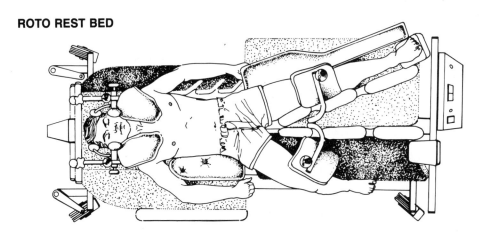

# ☐ Skull Tongs

### Purpose

To immobilize the spine and maintain vertebral alignment, which prevents cord damage from unstable bone fragments or misaligned vertebrae.

### Description

Commonly used tongs include Crutchfield, Gardner-Wells, and Vinke. They are inserted by a doctor with the assistance of a nurse.

## SKULL TONGS

All three types of cervical tongs consist of a stainless steel body with a pin (about ⅛" [0.3 cm] in diameter with a sharp tip) attached at each end. The pins on *Crutchfield tongs* are placed about 5" (12.7 cm) apart in line with the long axis of the cervical spine. The pins on the *Gardner-Wells tongs* are farther apart, with the pins inserted slightly above the patient's ears. The pins on *Vinke tongs* are placed at the parietal bones, near the widest transverse diameter of the skull, about 1" (2.54 cm) above the helix.

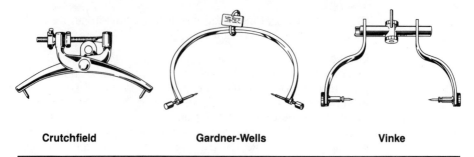

| Crutchfield | Gardner-Wells | Vinke |

*Crutchfield* or *Vinke tongs.* The patient is usually placed on a turning frame or special bed. The pin sites are shaved, prepared, and infiltrated with a local anesthetic. Small incisions are made at the insertion sites with a scalpel, and openings are made in the outer table of the skull with a twist drill. The tongs are inserted and tightened.

*Gardner-Wells tongs.* The patient's hair is clipped, not shaved. Insertion sites are lower (above the ear). Areas are prepared and infiltrated with a local anesthetic. Points have sharp tips and are twisted into the skull until the spring-loaded point shows proper pressure.

### Interventions

Prepare tongs, tong tray, shave-prep tray, 2% lidocaine, gloves, linen saver pad (under head), and povidone-iodine solution. When tongs are inserted, assist as needed. Use cotton-tipped applicators soaked in hydrogen peroxide to cleanse pin sites every 4 hours. Rinse the sites with saline solution, using the same technique. Apply antibacterial ointment. Watch for swelling, redness, or drainage from pin sites, which may indicate infection.

If the tongs become loosened or dislodged, reassure the patient, immobilize his head with sandbags on each side, and notify a doctor. Determine if the patient has sustained any new motor or sensory losses as a result. While traction is reestablished and maintained, perform neurologic checks and continue these checks at least every 4 hours for 12 hours. Weights should always hang freely. The knot in the rope should not rest against a pulley because this diminishes the weight's traction.

## ☐ Splints

### Purpose
To help maintain a functional position of the hands and feet, especially in patients with spastic paralysis.

### Description
Light splints are usually molded from Duraplast, which can be remolded to relieve a pressure point or to improve the functional position of an extremity. Velcro straps hold the splints in position.

**HAND SPLINT**

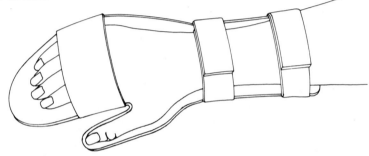

### Interventions
Check the splints for an appropriate fit. Alternate with hand rolls and footboard every 2 hours or apply 2 hours on, 2 hours off. Check the skin for reddened areas every 2 hours (readjust the splint if redness occurs), and perform range-of-motion exercises to wrists, fingers, ankles, and toes.

## ☐ Trochanter Roll

### Purpose
To prevent external hip rotation and maintain body alignment in the supine position.

### Description
In a supine position, the hip has a natural tendency toward external rotation. Wedging the lateral thigh with a rolled towel, trochanter roll, or foam wedge pad will keep the extremity in functional alignment and help prevent hip contracture.

## Interventions

A folded bath blanket may be used. Position the patient between rolls, and tighten them by turning downward until the hips are aligned. The roll should extend from the iliac crest to midthigh.

## TROCHANTER ROLL

A trochanter roll, illustrated at right, may be used to prevent external hip rotation and maintain body alignment.

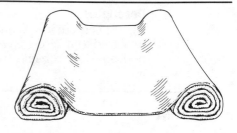

## TURNING YOUR PATIENT ON A STRYKER FRAME

### Frames and beds

To care for a patient with spinal cord injuries who's immobilized on a frame or bed, you'll need to know the following: how to maintain proper spinal alignment, how to prevent further spinal cord damage, and how to promote healing of his bony injury. Additionally, you must take measures to prevent skin breakdown and contracture deformities.

**Stryker frame**—A patient with severe neck or back injuries may be immobilized on a Stryker frame. Make sure you explain the purpose of the frame to your patient and his family; it will probably seem frightening to them. Unless your patient is prepared, he may fear falling when he's turned.

The Stryker frame uses an anterior and a posterior frame with canvas covers and thin padding over each. The frames, which are supported on a movable cart, have a pivot apparatus at each end. This allows you to change the patient's position to either prone or supine without altering his alignment.

To do this properly, follow the manufacturer's instructions or your hospital's procedure manual.

*Further tips:* Before turning your patient, secure any equipment he may have, such as I.V. lines, Foley catheter, or respirator tubing, to make sure it will turn easily with him.

Some patients prefer to be turned more quickly than others. Place your patient's pref-

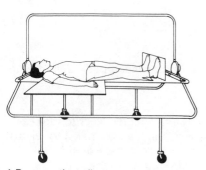

**1** Proper patient alignment *supine position*

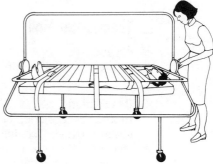

**2** Frame secured with safety straps over patient

# ☐ Turning Frames (Stryker, Foster)

## Purpose
To completely immobilize the spine.

## Description
A turning frame consists of two bed frames, which when secured in an anterior-posterior position, allow for lateral turning of the patient. Alignment and traction are maintained throughout the procedure.

Several companies make turning frames, so be sure to follow the manufacturer's instructions as well as your hospital's routine procedure. Do not attempt this procedure without another experienced person assisting you.

erence on his care plan along with the turning schedule.
• To prevent malalignment, check the equipment periodically and tighten the lacing of the canvases.
• To protect your patient's skin, place a foam mattress or padding on both frames and cover it with sheepskin.
• To aid in maintaining proper alignment, use a footboard, hand roll, bolsters, and splints, as required.
• You may add arm rest wings to the frame at shoulder level. They'll permit your patient to rest his arms and will help maintain alignment.
• For meals, place the patient in prone position.

• For elimination, place him in supine position, with his bedpan under the opening in the canvas.
• When your patient's prone, carefully watch him for signs of respiratory problems. This position makes breathing more difficult.
• Help prevent your patient from feeling isolated, especially when he's prone. If he likes TV, place a set on the floor. Can he move his arms? He may wish to have books or hobbies on a tray under the frame.
• To care for a patient with skull tongs on a Stryker frame, always maintain traction, even when turning. During the turn, the nurse positioned at the patient's head will check pulley and weights.

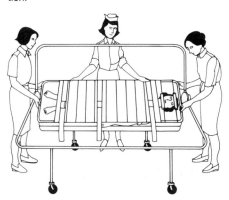

**3** Turning the patient

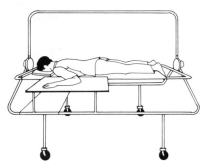

**4** Turn accomplished. Proper patient alignment *prone position*

### Interventions

General instructions for turning the supine patient include the following:
• Explain the procedure to the patient.
• Position I.V. lines, urinary catheters, chest tubes, and traction and other apparatus so that they don't become tangled during the turn.
• Remove the armboards and footboard.
• Place a pillow over the patient's thighs, and pad any other area where the skin is showing signs of possible breakdown.
• Make sure the patient's arms are straight at his sides.
• *With another person,* apply the top frame and secure the section with the nut and bolt.
• Strap the patient in the bed to prevent movement.
• After each person releases the stabilizing bolts at the head and foot of the bed, turn the frame simultaneously on the count of three.
• Release the frame bolts and remove the top frame.
• Check the patient's alignment, make sure he's comfortable, re-position tubing and other apparatus, and then replace the armboards.
• Turn the patient every 2 hours.
• Give pain medication before prone positioning if the patient requests it (prone positioning is uncomfortable for most patients).

## ☐ Wheelchair Transfer

### Procedure

To assist and teach the paraplegic patient to transfer from a bed to a wheelchair and back.

### Description

Teaching this transfer technique is a step-by-step process. Become thoroughly familiar with these steps before attempting to teach your patient, as shown at right.

### Interventions

• Pick a time when your patient is well rested to teach the transfer.
• Demonstrate the procedure to the patient, then stand by to assist him.
• One attempt is enough for an initial session.
• Return the patient to his bed and review the procedure, then allow him to rest.

## PATIENT TEACHING:
## HOW TO PERFORM A FORWARD-BACKWARD SITTING TRANSFER

Before you leave the hospital, your doctor wants you to learn how to get from your bed to your wheelchair. To learn how to do this transfer, follow these guidelines:

First, remove the wheelchair's leg rests. If they are not removable, swing them aside. Then, position the front of the wheelchair as close as possible to the side of your bed. Lock its wheels. If you cannot position the wheelchair yourself, ask someone to do it for you. The seat of the wheelchair should be facing the side of the bed.

Make sure you are sitting in bed with your legs extended.

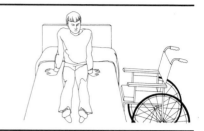

Next, lean slightly forward. Pushing your hands against the mattress, lift your buttocks slightly off the bed. Keeping your legs extended across the bed, inch backward to the side of the bed—close to the wheelchair. Stop when your back is directly in front of the wheelchair.

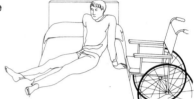

Now, firmly grasp the armrests of the wheelchair, and gradually lift your buttocks onto the seat. Unlock the wheels. Then, push yourself away from the bed, and position yourself properly in the wheelchair.

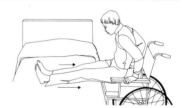

To get back into bed, position the wheelchair seat so that it faces the bed. Remove your legs from the leg rests. Then, swing the leg rests out of the way. Now, raise your legs onto the bed as you position the chair as close as possible to the bed. Lock the chair's wheels.

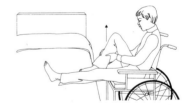

Next, grasp the armrests of the wheelchair, and lift your buttocks slightly off the seat. Keeping your legs extended across the bed, inch forward to the middle of the bed.

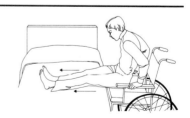

## ☐ Craniotomy

To access the brain for a surgical procedure, an opening must first be made in the skull; this is called a craniotomy. This procedure involves drilling four or five small burr holes and cutting the bone between them with a pneumatic drill or Gigli's wire saw. The bone remains attached to the muscle, which acts as a hinge when the flap is turned. In replacing the flap, some surgeons suture the bone flap to the skull with wire.

### Preoperative Care

Besides the routine preoperative care given to all surgical patients, the following special considerations apply to the neurosurgical patient:
• Explain the neurosurgical procedure to the patient and his family. Obtain signed consent form.
• Perform and record a preoperative neurologic assessment that includes level of consciousness, motor and sensory function, cranial nerve function, pupillary reaction, abnormal behavior, and a routine review of systems.
• Teach the patient postoperative leg exercises and deep breathing (vigorous coughing is contraindicated).
• Prepare the patient's scalp as ordered, usually with an antibacterial shampoo. Report any signs of infection or skin breaks. (The head is shaved in the operating room under general anesthesia.)
• Prepare the bowel as ordered. Instruct the patient to avoid straining at stool, both preoperatively and postoperatively, because this increases intracranial pressure (ICP).
• Tell the patient the approximate time the procedure will take place on the day of surgery.

### Immediate Preoperative Care

• Restrict food or fluids after midnight.
• Remove jewelry, and tape rings.
• Apply antiembolism stockings.
• Remove glasses, false teeth, and prosthetic devices.
• Record I.V. fluids given.
• Administer preoperative medications as ordered and document them.

## Postoperative Care

• Establish and maintain adequate airway and ventilation. Poor ventilation (particularly increased carbon dioxide in the blood) increases ICP.

• Count respirations a full minute every 15 minutes for the first hour, then follow routine care for neurosurgical patients on your unit. Note the character, rate, pattern, and depth of respirations and any apneic episodes.

• Take arterial blood gas measurements when ventilatory problems are suspected. This will require the doctor's order.

• Hyperventilate and hyperoxygenate before suctioning.

• Do not perform nasal suction without an order.

• Assess other vital signs and perform neurologic checks every 15 minutes for the first hour; then follow routine postoperative care for neurosurgical patients on your unit, checking for:
  —level of consciousness or orientation
  —pupillary size, shape, reaction to light, equality, or deviation
  —motor response changes
  —sensory response changes
  —any speech, behavioral, or vision changes not present at the preoperative examination.

• Take no oral temperatures with glass thermometers (patients may have seizures after surgery from irritated brain tissue).

• Maintain body alignment after supratentorial (above the cerebellum) surgery by:
  —elevating the head of the bed 30 degrees
  —positioning the patient on his side or back
  —keeping pressure off the operative site for 8 hours
  —permitting no neck flexion (interferes with cerebral drainage).

• Maintain body alignment after infratentorial (below the cerebellum) surgery by:
  —keeping the head of the bed flat
  —keeping the patient off his back for 24 to 48 hours
  —repositioning the patient from side to side every 2 hours while keeping his head in alignment.

• Assess surgical dressings for:
  —cerebrospinal fluid (CSF) leakage by looking for a light ring around dark drainage on a dressing (For nose and ear drainage, a positive Dextrostix test indicates probable CSF leakage.)
  —excessive bleeding.

• Record drainage from the wound drain on a flow sheet (empty every 4 hours).

• Implement seizure precautions.

• Restrain restless patients only on doctor's order.

• Use mitts if the patient pulls at I.V. lines or bothers the operative site.

• Put cool saline solution–soaked 4″ × 4″ gauze pads on the eyelids to reduce edema. Leave in place for about 15 minutes each hour, then replace with new pads at the next application. (Bacteria will grow beneath saline-soaked pads if they are reused or left on eyes for extended periods.)

• Administer all fluids by an infusion pump to avoid accidental fluid overload.

### Complications to report

• excessive restlessness
• seizure activity
• hypothermia or hyperthermia
• severe headache not relieved by analgesics
• sudden onset of a motor or sensory deficit or a change in the patient's level of consciousness or orientation
• pupillary changes

## ☐ Pituitary Surgery (Transsphenoidal Hypophysectomy)

Pituitary surgery may be approached through the sphenoidal sinus (as opposed to a craniotomy) to remove tumors. The incision is along the internal portion of the nasal septum, so the patient will return from surgery with a bandage over the nares.

The posterior pituitary stores antidiuretic hormone (ADH) and is sometimes damaged in surgery. Patients often will experience temporary diabetes insipidus (from a lack of ADH) postoperatively. Signs and symptoms of diabetes insipidus include excessive urination, dilute urine (a specific gravity of 1.001 to 1.006), and excessive thirst.

The nurse should check the nasal dressing for signs of CSF drainage or excessive bleeding. All previously mentioned neurologic evaluations apply to patients undergoing pituitary surgery.

## ☐ Spinal Surgery

The three most common spinal surgeries are laminectomies, spinal fusion, and cordotomy.

**Laminectomy** involves the partial removal of a herniated spinal disk's lamina.

**Spinal fusion** is a surgical procedure to solidify several vertebrae by grafting bone from a patient donor site to the lamina of the disks to be fused.

**Cordotomy** is a surgical procedure performed to divide the spinothalamic tract as a means of relieving intractable pain.

## Preoperative Care

• Stress the importance of positioning after surgery for correct body alignment.
• Teach the patient deep-breathing and range-of-motion exercises and the logroll technique.
• Explain postoperative drains, braces, special beds, and other equipment.
• Evaluate and record motor and sensory functions in all extremities.
• Record the type and extent of bowel or bladder dysfunction, if any.

## Immediate Preoperative Care

• Restrict food or fluids after midnight.
• Scrub the operative site with povidone-iodine solution; report any rashes or skin irritations.
• Apply antiembolism stockings.
• Insert a urinary catheter.
• Administer a cleansing enema.
• Start I.V. infusion and record amounts.
• Administer preoperative medications as ordered.

## Postoperative Care

• Provide bed rest with correct spinal alignment.
• Use the logroll technique when turning the patient. (Patient may arrive from O.R. on turning frame.)
• Check vital signs at least every hour for the first 4 hours, then routinely for neurosurgical patients on your unit.
• Check the dressing for drainage of blood and CSF.
• Perform neurologic checks, paying particular attention to movement of extremities and motor and sensory deficits.
• Compare the results of each neurologic check with the preoperative assessment.
• Perform range-of-motion exercises to extremities only if ordered.

# 6 | Neurologic Emergencies and Trauma

Traumatic emergencies frequently involve penetrating or blunt head injuries or problems involving vertebral misalignment and spinal cord compression or dissection. Other neurologic emergencies include coma of unknown etiology, generalized motor seizures, and myasthenic crisis.

The following neurologic emergencies are arranged in alphabetical order.

## ☐ Coma, Sudden Onset

On a general neurologic or neurosurgical unit, where patients are routinely observed for neurologic changes, the sudden onset of coma is usually attributed to neurologic factors. Keep in mind, however, that other disorders, such as diabetes, or accidental drug overdose may also bring about loss of consciousness.

The sudden onset of coma is an ominous sign indicating deterioration of the reticular activating system (RAS), which is part of the brain stem. The RAS is responsible for alertness; the brain stem, for vital life processes, including respiration and blood pressure. A patient's life is threatened when brain stem damage occurs.

### Interventions
• Establish and maintain a patent airway.
  —Insert an oropharyngeal airway immediately; prepare to intubate if ventilatory problems develop; administer oxygen at 8 liters/minute until the doctor arrives.
  —Place the patient on his side and suction his mouth, if necessary, to clear the airway.
• Perform a neurologic assessment, evaluating:
  —pupils (size, shape, equality, reaction to light, and deviation)
  —vital signs
  —Glasgow Coma Scale (for depth of coma, see *Assessing Level of Consciousness Using the Glasgow Coma Scale*).
• Expect the doctor to:
  —perform a neurologic examination
  —obtain arterial blood gas (ABG) measurements and intubate if impaired ventilation is clinically apparent
  —place the patient on a cardiac monitor
  —rule out a seizure by considering a history of onset, tongue biting, or incontinence
  —rule out hypoglycemia by determining serum glucose level

## ASSESSING LEVEL OF CONSCIOUSNESS USING THE GLASGOW COMA SCALE

To assess a patient's level of consciousness quickly in an emergency, use the Glasgow Coma Scale. Below you'll find an expanded version of this useful—though not compre- hensive—assessment technique. (A patient scoring 7 or less is comatose and probably has severe neurologic damage.)

| Test | Score | Patient's response |
|---|---|---|
| **Verbal response (when you ask, "What year is this?")** | | |
| Oriented | 5 | He tells you the current year. |
| Confused | 4 | He tells you an incorrect year. |
| Inappropriate words | 3 | He replies randomly: "tomorrow" or "roses." |
| Incomprehensible | 2 | He moans or screams. |
| None | 1 | He gives no response. |
| **Eye opening response** | | |
| Spontaneously | 4 | He opens his eyes spontaneously. |
| To speech | 3 | He opens his eyes when you tell him to. |
| To pain | 2 | He opens his eyes only on painful stimulus (for example, application of pressure to bony ridge under eyebrow). |
| None | 1 | He doesn't open his eyes in response to any stimulus. |
| **Motor response** | | |
| Obeys | 6 | He shows you two fingers when you ask him to. |
| Localizes | 5 | He reaches toward a painful stimulus and tries to remove it. |
| Withdraws | 4 | He moves away from a painful stimulus. |
| Abnormal flexion | 3 | He assumes a decorticate posture (below). |
| Abnormal extension | 2 | He assumes a decerebrate posture (below). |
| None | 1 | He doesn't respond at all, just lies flaccid—an *ominous sign*. |

—rule out internal bleeding with a brief physical examination and by determining hemoglobin and hematocrit levels

—rule out accidental overdose with a drug screen (Emergency Admissions)

—rule out hypovolemia by determining hematocrit and blood pressure.

*Note:* Sudden loss of consciousness in neurologic or neurosurgical patients is frequently caused by increased intracranial pressure (ICP) from hemorrhage, edema, injury, or other space-occupying lesions in the brain. This results in compression and herniation of areas that sustain consciousness and renders the patient comatose.

# ☐ Head Injuries, Closed

Closed (or blunt) head injuries are nonpenetrating wounds caused by striking the head against a solid object. The intracranial vault is not exposed to environmental contaminants. The three types of closed head injuries are:

• *coup* (pronounced "coo") injuries, which occur directly beneath the point of impact

• *contrecoup* injuries, which are caused by the brain rebounding against the skull opposite the impact site.

• *torsion* injuries, where the brain twists on its stem within the cranial vault. This "shearing" movement may produce cerebral edema in the uncal area. Herniation through the uncus or foramen magnum may occur following severe torsion injuries.

Blunt trauma requires close monitoring of neurologic status because, even though the patient shows no outward sign of major injury, he may nonetheless have sustained severe brain damage. Frequently encountered sequelae to blunt trauma include concussions and contusions.

**Concussion** results from an impact that causes temporary loss of consciousness but no visible brain damage on computed tomography (CT) scan or magnetic resonance imaging. Observe the patient especially for subtle changes in level of consciousness and signs and symptoms of increased ICP, as discussed on page 5.

**Contusion** results from an impact that produces actual brain injury (temporary or permanent bruising) that is usually visible on a CT scan. Observe the patient for changes in level of consciousness and signs and symptoms of increased ICP.

**Hemorrhage** may result from laceration of cerebral vessels or from shearing forces. Patients with hemorrhage (or developing hematoma) behave similarly to those with a rapidly developing space-occupying lesion. They should be monitored closely for signs of increasing ICP.

## INTRACRANIAL HEMATOMA: OCCUPYING SPACE AND INCREASING PRESSURE

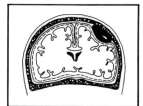 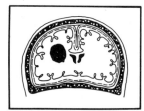 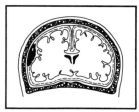

**Epidural hematoma**
Laceration of middle meningeal artery or vein, often resulting from a fracture, is the most common source of bleeding. But bleeding may also result from a tear in a dural sinus.

**Intracerebral hematoma**
Cerebral contusion is a common cause.

**Subdural hematoma**
Bleeding usually occurs from a torn bridging vein or cortical vessel or (less commonly) from a ruptured saccular aneurysm or an intracerebral hemorrhage.

 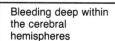 

Bleeding between the skull and dura mater into the epidural space

Bleeding deep within the cerebral hemispheres

Bleeding between the arachnoid membrane and the dura mater in the subdural space
*Acute* within 48 hours
*Subacute* from 2 days to 2 weeks
*Chronic* over 2 weeks

 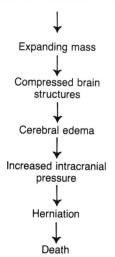

Expanding mass

↓

Compressed brain structures

↓

Cerebral edema

↓

Increased intracranial pressure

↓

Herniation

↓

Death

**Cerebral edema** is thought to be caused by a combination of cerebrovascular congestion and increased fluid accumulation in the injured area. Brain tissue damage can result from acceleration or deceleration injuries, which can cause shearing or torsion (stretching and twisting) of the brain stem that results in swelling.

Since the brain stem controls vital functions, this type of injury is critical and requires constant neurologic observation. The top priority in caring for these patients is close monitoring of brain stem function with frequent cranial nerve checks and pupillary observation as well as checking for other signs and symptoms of increased ICP.

# ☐ Head Injuries, Open

Open head injuries involve a penetration or break in the skull that exposes the brain to infection. Such injuries tend to be accompanied by dural tears, cerebral tissue injury, or hemorrhage. The risk of infection is a major complication. The three most common types of open head injuries are listed below.

**Depressed skull fractures.** Inward depression of bone fragments to at least the skull's thickness may occur, and some may penetrate the dura.

**Comminuted fractures.** Bone fragments may become imbedded in brain tissue.

**Missile injuries.** Bullets or other projectiles may remain imbedded or may create a destructive path through brain tissue, leaving entrance and exit wounds in the skull.

## Dangers of Open Injuries

• meningeal infection
• laceration of brain tissue
• leakage of cerebrospinal fluid (CSF).

*Note:* Basilar skull fractures often involve transverse injury to the perinasal sinuses, through which the brain may become infected via the nares. Patients with this injury should have nasal drainage checked for CSF leakage. Look for dark drainage surrounded by a light area on the dressing. If the light area tests positive with a Dextrostix, the drainage is probably CSF.

## Treatment

Open injuries require prompt surgical intervention to elevate depressed fractures and remove foreign objects. This relieves brain pressure and irritation. Such measures as restricting fluids, tilting the head of the bed 30 degrees, and administering dexamethasone (Decadron) are tried before surgery to reduce brain swelling.

## Interventions

Postoperative care of the patient with an open head wound is the same as that for a craniotomy. Since the risk of infection is higher, patients with head injuries should be monitored closely for meningeal signs (see page 63).

# ☐ Myasthenic Crisis

Two types of crises exist in myasthenia gravis: cholinergic and myasthenic. To differentiate them, the Tensilon test is performed. Edrophonium chloride (Tensilon) is administered intravenously, and the patient's response is observed. If signs and symptoms worsen, the crisis is cholinergic. If muscle strength improves, the crisis is myasthenic.

Both myasthenic and cholinergic crises produce similar signs and symptoms. However, different medical treatments are necessary because of their different causes.

## Signs and Symptoms
• history of myasthenia gravis
• respiratory insufficiency (from weakened respiratory muscles)
• difficulty speaking
• difficulty swallowing
• decreased gag reflex
• increased salivation

## Interventions
• Ensure adequate ventilation.
  —Expect to intubate if respiratory failure is imminent.
  —Check ABG levels (respiratory failure is defined as $PaO_2 <$ 50 mm HG and $PaCO_2 > 50$ mm Hg).
• Be prepared to suction the patient as needed.
• Be prepared to administer an anticholinesterase I.V. for myasthenic crisis.
• Be prepared to administer atropine I.V. for cholinergic crisis.
• Place the patient on a cardiac monitor.
  *Note:* Check your patient's medication orders before administering the following drugs that exacerbate myasthenic crisis:
• barbiturates
• narcotics
• antianxiety agents
• quinidine
• procainamide
• aminoglycoside antibiotics (streptomycin, gentamicin, and neomycin).

## ☐ Seizures and Status Epilepticus
### Generalized Tonic-Clonic Status Epilepticus
Status epilepticus is defined as a continuous tonic-clonic seizure activity without complete recovery between seizures.

### Signs and Symptoms
• unconsciousness
• continuous tonic-clonic seizure activity
• sustained deviation of eyes
• incontinence
• diaphoresis
• labored breathing
• apneic episodes
• cyanosis

### Interventions
• Maintain adequate oxygenation (as much as possible) while medically treating the patient.
• Hypoxia is the greatest physiologic danger of status epilepticus. Brain damage and death may ensue if oxygen is not supplied.
  —Turn the patient's head to the side and suction if necessary during less active intervals.
  —Check ABG measurements when possible.
  —Provide oxygen at 8 to 10 liters/minute.
  —Expect to assist with endotracheal intubation during the partial recovery phase; the nasal route may be attempted.
• Protect the patient from injury.
  —Hold his head and lower him to the floor if the patient was standing during onset.
  —Administer anticonvulsants, such as diazepam (Valium), by I.V. push, usually ordered two or three times at 20-minute intervals. Anticonvulsant medications commonly used besides diazepam include phenytoin (Dilantin), phenobarbital, and paraldehyde.
• Expect to insert a nasogastric tube once the patient is intubated.
  *Note:* Prolonged seizure activity results in hypoxia, hypoglycemia, and hyperthermia. These conditions, in turn, contribute to further seizure activity, resulting in metabolic or physical exhaustion, and even death, if not treated.

### Seizure Precautions
Patients susceptible to brain tissue irritation, such as those with epilepsy or head injuries, are prone to seizures. The following

guidelines ensure maximum safety for these patients:
- Tape a soft oral airway or rolled washcloth on the headboard. Airways can be inserted during an aura that may precede a seizure but are never inserted once the seizure has started.
- Place the patient in a carpeted room if possible.
- Keep the bed in a low position.
- Keep the side rails padded and up while the patient is in bed.
- Prohibit unsupervised smoking.
- Provide a quiet environment.
- Take no oral temperatures with glass thermometers.
- Provide patients with their own room for privacy if possible.

## Classification of Seizures

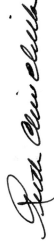

Seizures are classified primarily as partial or generalized. (See *Differentiating between Seizure Types,* pages 118 and 119.) They are caused by brain tissue irritation that may be idiopathic or may result from injury, surgery, or a space-occupying lesion.

### Partial seizures

Partial seizures occur without loss of consciousness. The classification is divided into simple seizures (such as focal motor and Jacksonian) and complex seizures, which involve various dyscognitive states.

*Auras* are states of altered consciousness that often precede focal seizures. These periods may last from a few seconds to 4 or 5 minutes. During this time, the patient has a blank stare and may experience psychosensory or psychomotor hallucinations, such as foul smells and tastes, vertigo, and unfamiliarity with the environment. If the patient can familiarize himself with the onset of these feelings and sensations, he can seek a relatively safe place before the seizure begins.

### Generalized seizures

Generalized seizures present with loss of consciouness. They are usually tonic-clonic seizures characterized by incontinence, excessive salivation, and postictal weakness and lethargy. Variations include absence seizures and myoclonic and akinetic attacks.

## Nursing Observations

- Before the seizure (preictal phase), check for:
  - —level of consciousness
  - —activity before attack
  - —portion of the body in which the seizure starts.

*(continued on page 120)*

## DIFFERENTIATING BETWEEN SEIZURE TYPES

| Disorder | Areas involved (focus) | Change in consciousness |
|---|---|---|
| *Partial seizures (simple)* | | |
| **Focal motor** | Motor strip on precentral gyrus in frontal lobe | Unilateral: No change in consciousness. Bilateral: Loss of consciousness. |
| **Jacksonian** | Motor strip on precentral gyrus in frontal lobe | Unilateral: No change in consciousness. Bilateral: Loss of consciousness. |
| **Adversive** | Frontal lobe anterior to motor strip | No loss |
| **Epilepsia partialis continua** | Varied | No loss |
| **Focal sensory** | Postcentral gyrus in parietal or occipital lobe | No loss |
| *Partial seizures (complex)* | | |
| **Psychomotor** | Temporal lobe | No loss of consciousness; confusion and amnesia |
| *Generalized seizures* | | |
| **Generalized tonic-clonic (grand mal)** | Generalized | Loss of consciousness with postictal sleeping |
| **Absence (petit mal)** | Generalized | Transient losses of consciousness; no postictal state |
| **Infantile spasms** | Generalized | None; no postictal state |
| **Myoclonic** | Generalized | Possible momentary loss of consciousness followed by confusion |
| **Akinetic (drop attacks)** | Generalized, with brain stem involvement | None; no postictal state |
| *Miscellaneous* | | |
| **Mixed** | Frontal, temporal, or occipital focus with generalized spread | Consistent with type of seizure |

| EEG findings | Impaired capacities |
|---|---|
| Focal waves, slow waves, or spikes | Convulsive movements and temporary disturbance in motor capacity in body part controlled by that brain region |
| Focal waves, slow waves, or spikes | Disturbance in motor capacity. Seizure activity marches along limb or side of body in orderly progression. |
| Focal waves, slow waves, or spikes | Disturbance in behavior and motor capacity. Head and eyes turn away from focal region. May develop into generalized seizure. |
| Focal waves, slow waves, or spikes | Form of local status epilepticus involving muscle group. May last minutes to weeks with postictal weakness. |
| Spikes and slow waves over epileptogenic focus in occipital or parietal areas | Subjective sensory experience; may be visual, auditory, olfactory, or somatosensory. Possible "marching" progression. |
| Temporal spikes or slow waves | Hallucinations, dyscognitive states (déjà vu), automatism, and loss of awareness |
| Rapidly repeating spikes in tonic phase; spikes or slow waves in clonic phase | Major tonic muscular contraction followed by longer phase of clonic (jerking) contractions. Possible bowel and bladder incontinence, weakness, injury, or learning disorders. |
| Spikes and waves, three/second | Interference with conscious response to environment when uncontrolled; possible learning disorders |
| Multiple spikes and slow waves of large amplitude (hypsarrhythmia) | Jackknife, flexor spasms of extremities and head. Severe mental and developmental deficiencies. |
| Findings similar to those for infantile spasms | Uncontrollable jerking movements of extremities or entire body |
| Normal to slow background with polyspike or multiple spike waves | Sudden postural tone loss. Possible intellectual, perceptual, and motor impairment. |
| Spike, polyspike, or spike-wave patterns with progression of focus to a generalized pattern | Interferences with behavior, learning, or motor functions |

• During the seizure (interictal phase), check for:
—the patient crying out
—automatisms (eye fluttering or lip smacking)
—bilateral movements
—length of seizure
—salivation
—cyanosis
—incontinence
—pupil activity.
• After the seizure (postictal phase), check for:
—lethargy
—confusion
—headache
—speech impairment
—other neurologic deficits, such as transient hemiplegia.

### Interventions
• Support the patient's head.
• Lower the patient to the floor if he was standing at the seizure's onset.
• Insert a soft oral airway if the full onset of seizures has not begun.
• Maintain a patent airway and oxygenation.
• Observe and report the event as described on page 54.
• Administer medications as ordered.
• Reorient the patient after the seizure.
• Perform a neurologic assessment after the seizure.

## ☐ Spinal Injuries
Spinal cord trauma, caused by misaligned or fractured vertebrae, consists of four types of injury: compression, complete or partial transection, bruising, or irritation. One danger in this type of injury is that spinal movements can cause additional injuries and permanent damage (if this hasn't already occurred).

In multiple trauma and head injury, possible spinal trauma is always suspected. In the field as well as in the hospital, *spinal immobilization* is the most important aspect of patient care after airway maintenance and restoration of breathing and cardiac function.

*Note:* For an emergency airway, the triple airway or jaw-thrust maneuver is employed, so that cervical spine alignment is not disturbed. Endotracheal intubation, if required, is initially attempted nasally (blind intubation). Cervical spine X-rays are among the first procedures performed when the patient arrives in the emergency department.

## WHAT HAPPENS IN SPINAL CORD INJURY

**Traumatic spinal lesions** (such as contusions, lacerations, vertebral fractures, or hemorrhages) disrupt the intercommunication of the patient's spinal cord, brain, and the rest of his body. The injury may cause loss of both voluntary and autonomic motor activity. The lesion's location (cervical, thoracic, lumbar, or sacral) and the type and extent of cord injury determine how much motor and sensory function the patient loses.

Types of spinal cord injuries include flexion-rotation, hyperextension, compression, and penetration injuries. Here's what you should know about how these types of spinal cord injuries occur.

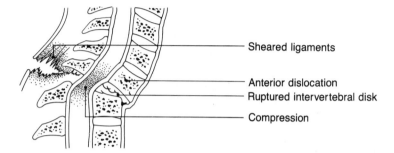

Sheared ligaments

Anterior dislocation
Ruptured intervertebral disk

Compression

**Flexion injury** frequently involves the cervical and lumbar spine. This type of injury generally results from impact to the posterior fossa that propels the patient's neck onto his chest, causing anterior dislocation, a ruptured intervertebral disk, or, possibly, a fractured pedicle, vertebral body, or wedge fracture. With any vertebral fracture, if the ligamentous support to the vertebral column is also disrupted, the spinal cord's stability and integrity are jeopardized.

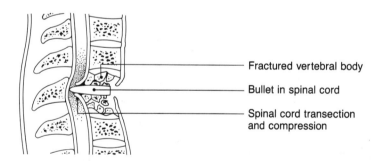

Fractured vertebral body

Bullet in spinal cord

Spinal cord transection
and compression

**Penetration injury** occurs when a penetrating object shatters a vertebral body or the ligamentous support on entry to the patient's spinal canal. Spinal cord tissue is damaged or transected, causing hemorrhage, compression, and infarction. In penetration injuries, as in all types of spinal cord injuries, edema may result from trauma, causing further compression above and below the level of injury.

*(continued)*

## WHAT HAPPENS IN SPINAL CORD INJURY *(continued)*

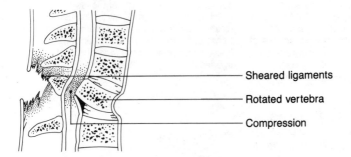

— Sheared ligaments

— Rotated vertebra

— Compression

**Flexion-rotation injury** occurs when the patient's head and body are twisted in opposite directions, dislocating cervical vertebrae and shearing supporting ligaments. The resulting vertebral malalignment compresses the spinal column.

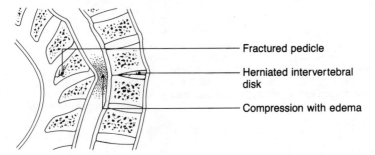

— Fractured pedicle

— Herniated intervertebral disk

— Compression with edema

**Hyperextension injury** occurs when the patient's head is thrown back sharply, disrupting various supporting ligaments, rupturing intervertebral disks, and fracturing one or more vertebral bodies or pedicles. This compresses the patient's spine and makes it unstable.

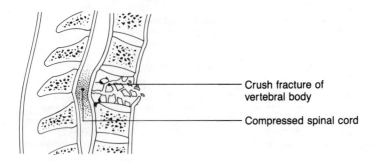

— Crush fracture of vertebral body

— Compressed spinal cord

**Compression injury** results from a vertical force to the top of the patient's head or from an upward force to his feet, often due to a fall from an extreme height. This causes a crush fracture of a vertebral body with impingement on the cord or nerve roots.

## Early management of spinal injuries
• dexamethasone (Decadron) to control edema, usually 4 mg I.V., four to six times daily
• immobilization
  —For cervical injuries, skull tongs or skeletal traction may be used (see pages 99 to 100).
  —For thoracic or lumbar injuries, a halo device with femoral traction may be used. Steinmann pins are inserted into the distal end of both femurs and attached to the halo with adjustable rods (see page 91).
  —For more extensive injuries, a body cast may be used. The patient receives cast care with special attention to hygiene and prevention of pressure sores. Logrolling must be used when moving the patient.

## Interventions
Medical treatment involves surgery to fuse or align vertebrae or to remove bone fragments that pose a threat of cord injury. For postoperative care, see page 109.

### UNDERSTANDING MOTOR AND SENSORY IMPAIRMENT IN COMPLETE SPINAL CORD INJURY

| Area affected | | Type of motor loss | Area of sensory loss (pain, temperature, touch, and pressure) |
|---|---|---|---|
| Cervical nerve roots | C1 to C4 | • Diaphragm paresis • Intercostal paralysis • Flaccid total paralysis in skeletal muscles below neck | • Neck and below |
| | C5 to C8 | • Intercostal paralysis • Paralysis below shoulders and upper arms | • Arms and hands, chest, abdomen, and lower extremities |
| Thoracic nerve roots | T1 to T6 | • Paralysis below midchest | • Below midchest |
| | T7 to T12 | • Paralysis below waist | • Below waist |
| Lumbar nerve roots | L1 to L3 | • Paralysis in most leg muscles and in pelvis | • Lower abdomen and legs |
| | L4 to L5 | • Paralysis in lower legs, ankles, and feet | • Parts of lower legs and feet |
| Sacral nerve roots | S1 to S5 | • Ataxic paralysis of the bladder and rectum • Paralysis of feet and ankles | • Posterior inner thigh, lateral foot, and perineum |

# 7 Neurologic drugs

The following neurologic drugs are arranged in alphabetical order by classification.

## NEUROLOGIC DRUGS

| Drug, dosage, and route | Interactions | Adverse reactions | Special considerations |
|---|---|---|---|
| *Anticonvulsants* | | | |
| **acetazolamide** 375 mg to 1 g P.O. daily in divided doses | *Ephedrine, pseudoephedrine:* increased central nervous system (CNS) stimulation. *Lithium:* decreased therapeutic effects. *Methenamine:* antagonized methenamine effect. | Aplastic anemia, hyperchloremic acidosis | Obtain complete blood count (CBC) and serum electrolyte levels every 3 months. Also, drug is usually given with other anticonvulsants. Monitor for hyperglycemia in prediabetics or diabetics on insulin or oral drugs. |
| **carbamazepine** 800 mg to 1.2 g P.O. daily in divided doses | *Nicotinic acid:* may decrease carbamazepine levels. Monitor for lack of therapeutic effect. *Propoxyphene:* may increase carbamazepine levels. Use another analgesic. *Troleandomycin, erythromycin, isoniazid:* may increase carbamazepine blood levels. Use together cautiously. | Blood dyscrasias, dizziness, drowsiness, ataxia, nausea, stomatitis, dry mouth | May cause mild-to-moderate dizziness when first taken. Effect usually disappears within 4 days. Obtain CBC and platelet count weekly for first 3 months, then monthly. Tell patient to notify doctor immediately if fever, sore throat, mouth ulcers, or easy bruising occurs. When used for trigeminal neuralgia, an attempt should be made every 3 months to decrease dose or to stop drug. |
| **clonazepam** 0.5 to 2 mg P.O. t.i.d. | None significant. | Drowsiness, ataxia, increased salivation | Warn patient to avoid activities that require alertness and good psychomotor coordination until CNS response to drug has been determined. Never withdraw drug suddenly. Tell patient to report side effects immediately. Also monitor patient for oversedation. |
| **diazepam** *For status epilepticus:* 5 to 20 mg by slow I.V. push; may repeat q 5 | None significant. | Cardiovascular collapse, drowsiness, ataxia, pain at injection site, thrombophlebitis | Don't mix with other drugs or I.V. fluids. Avoid storing in plastic syringe or infusing through plastic tubing. Infuse at rate not exceed- |

## NEUROLOGIC DRUGS *(continued)*

| Drug, dosage, and route | Interactions | Adverse reactions | Special considerations |
|---|---|---|---|
| *Anticonvulsants* | | | |
| **diazepam** *(continued)* to 10 minutes to maximum dose of 60 mg | | | ing 5 mg/minute and preferably at 2 mg/minute to decrease risk of respiratory depression and hypotension. Monitor respirations every 5 to 15 minutes and before each repeated dose. Have emergency resuscitative equipment and oxygen at bedside. Also watch for phlebitis at injection site. |
| **ethosuximide** 20 mg/kg P.O. in divided doses; maximum dose— 1.5 g daily | None significant. | Nausea, vomiting, anorexia, epigastric distress, drowsiness, euphoria, dizziness, blood dyscrasias | Warn patient to avoid activities that require alertness and good psychomotor coordination until CNS response to drug has been determined. Obtain CBC every 3 months. Never withdraw drug suddenly. |
| **ethotoin** 2 to 3 g P.O. daily in divided doses | *Alcohol, folic acid, loxapine:* decreased ethotoin activity. *Oral anticoagulants, antihistamines, chloramphenicol, diazepam, diazoxide, disulfiram, isoniazid, phenylbutazone, salicylates, valproate:* increased ethotoin activity and toxicity. | Nausea, vomiting, diarrhea, lymphadenopathy | Give after meals. Schedule doses as evenly as possible over 24 hours. Stop drug at once if lymphadenopathy or lupus-like syndrome develops. Hydantoin derivative of choice in young adults who are prone to gingival hyperplasia caused by phenytoin. Otherwise, it's infrequently used for treating epilepsy. |
| **mephenytoin** 200 to 600 mg P.O. daily in three divided doses | *Alcohol, folic acid, loxapine:* decreased mephenytoin activity. *Oral anticoagulants, antihistamines, chloramphenicol, diazepam, diazoxide, disulfiram, isoniazid, phenylbutazone, salicylates, valproate:* increased mephenytoin activity and toxicity. | Drowsiness, blood dyscrasias, skin rash, exfoliative dermatitis | Tell patient to notify doctor if fever, sore throat, bleeding, or skin rash occurs. These signs may indicate serious blood dyscrasias. Check CBC and platelet count initially and every 2 weeks thereafter, up to 2 weeks after full dose attained; then monthly. Stop drug if neutrophil count falls below 1,600/mm$^3$. |
| **mephobarbital** 400 to 600 mg P.O. daily in single or divided doses | Monoamine oxidase (MAO) inhibitors: *potentiate barbiturate effect.* Oral anticoagulants: | Dizziness, drowsiness, lethargy, skin eruptions | Warn patient to avoid activities that require alertness and good psychomotor coordination *(continued)* |

## NEUROLOGIC DRUGS *(continued)*

| Drug, dosage, and route | Interactions | Adverse reactions | Special considerations |
|---|---|---|---|
| *Anticonvulsants* | | | |
| **mephobarbital** *(continued)* | *possible decreased anti-coagulant effect.* *Rifampin:* may decrease barbiturate levels. Monitor for decreased effect. | | until CNS response to drug has been determined. Store drug in light-resistant container. In adults, give total or largest dose at night if seizures occur then. Warn patient to use drug cautiously with alcohol, narcotics, or other CNS depressants. |
| **paraldehyde** *For status epilepticus:* 5 to 10 ml I.M.; 0.2 to 0.4 ml/kg in 0.9% saline solution by I.V. injection | *Alcohol:* increased CNS depression. Use together cautiously. *Disulfiram:* increased paraldehyde blood levels; possible toxic disulfiram reaction. Use together cautiously. | Pulmonary edema or hemorrhage, circulatory collapse (from I.V. use), foul breath odor, skin rash | Divide 10-ml I.M. dose into two injections. Inject deeply, away from nerve trunks, and massage injection site. Use glass syringe and bottle for parenteral dose since drug reacts with plastic. Don't use if solution is brown or has a vinegary odor, or if container has been open longer than 24 hours. |
| **paramethadione** 0.9 to 2.4 g P.O. daily in three or four divided doses | None significant. | Blood dyscrasias, drowsiness, exfoliative dermatitis, skin rash, photophobia | Tell patient to immediately report sore throat, fever, malaise, bruises, petechiae, or epistaxis. Advise him to wear dark glasses if photophobia occurs. |
| **phenobarbital** *For status epilepticus:* 10 mg/kg by I.V. infusion no faster than 50 mg/minute; maximum dose—20 mg/kg *For epilepsy:* usual maintenance dose—100 to 200 mg P.O. daily in single or divided doses | *Alcohol and other CNS depressants, including narcotic analgesics:* excessive CNS depression. *MAO inhibitors:* potentiated barbiturate effect. *Oral anticoagulants:* possible decreased anticoagulant effect. *Rifampin:* may decrease barbiturate levels. Monitor for decreased effect. | Lethargy, drowsiness, hangover, skin eruptions | Reserve I.V. injection for emergency treatment, and give slowly under close supervision. Monitor respirations carefully. Watch for signs of barbiturate toxicity: asthmatic breathing, cyanosis, clammy skin, hypotension, coma. Overdose can be fatal. Don't use injection solution if it contains a precipitate. |
| **phensuximide** 500 mg to 1 g P.O. b.i.d. or t.i.d. | None significant. | Nausea, vomiting, drowsiness, dizziness | Never withdraw drug suddenly; this may cause petit mal seizures. Report side effects immediately. Drug may cause pink, red, or reddish-brown urine. |

## NEUROLOGIC DRUGS *(continued)*

| Drug, dosage, and route | Interactions | Adverse reactions | Special considerations |
|---|---|---|---|
| **Anticonvulsants** | | | |
| **phenytoin** *For status epilepticus:* 500 mg to 1 g I.V. at 50 mg/ minute. *For epilepsy:* maintenance dose— 300 to 600 mg P.O. daily or in divided doses | *Alcohol, folic acid, loxapine:* decreased phenytoin activity. *Oral anticoagulants, antihistamines, chloramphenicol, cimetidine, diazepam, diazoxide, disulfiram, isoniazid, phenylbutazone, salicylates, thioridazine, valproate:* phenytoin toxicity risk. | Nausea, vomiting, gingival hyperplasia, blood dyscrasias, rash, exfoliative dermatitis, hirsutism, nystagmus, diplopia, blurred vision, drowsiness, dizziness, confusion, hallucinations, slurred speech | Give divided doses with or after meals to decrease GI side effects. Stop drug if skin rash appears. If rash is scarlet or measles-like, resume drug after rash clears. If rash reappears, stop drug. If rash is exfoliative purpuric, or bullous, don't resume drug. Provide patient with instructions. Use only clear solution for injection. Consider slight yellowing acceptable. Don't refrigerate drug. |
| **primidone** 250 mg P.O. t.i.d. or q.i.d. | *Carbamazepine:* increased primidone levels. Observe for toxicity. *Phenytoin:* stimulates conversion of primidone to phenobarbital. Observe for increased phenobarbital effect. | Drowsiness, diplopia, lethargy, nausea, vomiting | Warn patient to avoid activities that require alertness and good psychomotor coordination until CNS response to drug has been determined. Drug is partially converted to phenobarbital by body metabolism. Shake liquid suspension well. |
| **valproic acid valproate sodium** 15 to 30 mg/kg daily, usually in divided doses | *Antacids, aspirin:* may cause valproic acid toxicity. Use together cautiously and monitor blood levels. | Nausea, vomiting, indigestion, thrombocytopenia, hepatotoxicity | Obtain liver function studies, platelet count, and prothrombin time before starting drug and every month thereafter. Nonspecific symptoms, such as fever and lethargy, may signal severe hepatotoxicity. |
| **Anti-infectives** | | | |
| **cefotaxime** 1 g I.V. or I.M. q 6 to 8 hours; maximum dose—12 g daily in life-threatening infections | *Probenecid:* may inhibit excretion and increase blood levels of cefotaxime. | Diarrhea, pseudomembranous colitis, rash, urticaria, pain at injection site, thrombophlebitis (with I.V. administration) | Give drug I.V. rather than I.M. in life-threatening infection. When administering I.M., inject deep into a large muscle mass, such as the gluteus or lateral aspect of thigh. |

*(continued)*

## NEUROLOGIC DRUGS (continued)

| Drug, dosage, and route | Interactions | Adverse reactions | Special considerations |
|---|---|---|---|
| *Anti-infectives* | | | |
| **chloramphenicol** 50 to 100 mg/kg P.O. or I.V. daily in divided doses q 6 hours; maximum dose—100 mg/ kg daily | *Acetaminophen:* elevated chloramphenicol levels. *Oral anticoagulants:* possible bleeding. *Penicillins:* antagonized antibacterial effect. Give penicillin at least 1 hour before chloramphenicol. *Sulfonylureas:* increased hypoglycemia. | Aplastic anemia, granulocytopenia, dose-related anemia | Monitor CBC, platelet and reticulocyte counts, and serum iron levels before and every 2 days during therapy. Stop drug immediately if anemia, reticulocytopenia, leukopenia, or thrombocytopenia develops. |
| **moxalactam** 2 to 6 g I.V. or I.M. daily in divided doses q 8 hours; maximum dose—12 g daily in life-threatening infections | *Ethyl alcohol:* may cause disulfiram-like reaction. Warn patient not to drink alcohol for several days after discontinuing moxalactam. | Hypoprothrombinemia with possible severe bleeding, diarrhea, pseudomembranous colitis, rash, urticaria, pain at injection site, thrombophlebitis | When administering I.M., inject deep into a large muscle mass, such as the gluteus or lateral aspect of thigh. If severe bleeding occurs after high doses, promptly give vitamin K. |
| **nafcillin** 2 to 12 g I.V. or I.M. daily in divided doses q 4 to 6 hours | *Aminoglycoside antibiotics:* separate I.V. nafcillin dose by at least 1 hour. Don't mix together in same I.V. container. *Chloramphenicol, erythromycin, tetracyclines:* antibiotic antagonism. Give nafcillin at least 1 hour before. *Probenecid:* increased blood levels of nafcillin. (Probenecid is often used for this purpose.) | Hypersensitivity, skin rash, thrombophlebitis | Before giving nafcillin, ask patient if he's had any allergic reactions to penicillin. Check drug's expiration date. Give intermittently I.V. to prevent vein irritation. Also change site every 48 hours. |
| **penicillin G** 1.2 to 24 million units I.M. or I.V. daily in divided doses q 4 hours | *Aminoglycoside antibiotics:* separate I.V. penicillin dose by at least 1 hour. Don't mix together in same I.V. container. *Chloramphenicol, erythromycin, tetracyclines:* antibiotic antagonism. Give penicillin at least 1 hour before bacteriostatic antibiotics. *Probenecid:* increased blood levels of penicillin. (Probenecid is often used for this purpose.) | Hypersensitivity, skin rash, thrombophlebitis | Before giving penicillin, ask the patient if he's had any allergic reactions to this drug. Check drug's expiration date. Give intermittently I.V. to prevent vein irritation. Also change site every 48 hours. Superinfection may occur with prolonged therapy, especially in elderly and debilitated patients. |

## NEUROLOGIC DRUGS *(continued)*

| Drug, dosage, and route | Interactions | Adverse reactions | Special considerations |
|---|---|---|---|
| *Antivirals* | | | |
| **acyclovir (parenteral)** 5 to 10 mg/kg q 8 hours for 7 to 10 days; give at constant rate over 1 hour | *Interferon or methotrexate (intrathecal):* may result in neurologic abnormalities | Phlebitis at injection site. Elevated serum creatinine, rash or hives. | Administer over a period of at least 1 hour to prevent renal damage. Check injection site frequently for extravasation of I.V. fluid. |
| **vidarabine** 15 mg/kg daily for 10 days; give by slow I.V. infusion over 12 to 24 hours | *Allopurinol:* increased incidence of CNS side effects. | Anorexia, nausea, tremor, dizziness, confusion | Don't give I.M. or S.C. because of low solubility and poor absorption. Administer with an in-line I.V. filter 0.45 micron or smaller. CNS side effects must be distinguished from symptoms of encephalitis. |
| *Antimyasthenics* | | | |
| **neostigmine** 15 to 30 mg P.O. t.i.d.; 0.5 to 2 mg I.M. or I.V. q 1 to 3 hours, as needed | *Procainamide, aminoglycoside antibiotics, quinidine:* may reverse cholinergic effect on muscle. Observe for lack of therapeutic effect. *Succinylcholine:* prolonged respiratory depression and possible apnea. | Nausea, vomiting, diarrhea, muscle cramps, respiratory depression | Monitor vital signs frequently, especially respirations. Keep atropine injection available to treat serious side effects. Give drug with milk or food to reduce GI side effects. Document patient's response after each dose. Show patient how to observe and record variations in muscle strength. |
| **pyridostigmine** 60 to 180 mg P.O. b.i.d. or q.i.d. with maximum dose of 1,500 mg; 2 mg I.M. or very slow I.V. injection q 3 hours | *Procainamide, aminoglycoside antibiotics, quinidine:* may reverse cholinergic effect on muscle. Observe for lack of therapeutic effect. *Succinylcholine:* prolonged respiratory depression and apnea. | Nausea, vomiting, diarrhea, headache | Parenteral dose is ⅓₀ of oral dose. Double-check all orders for I.M. or I.V. administration. Adjust dose depending on patient response. |
| *Antineoplastics* | | | |
| **carmustine (BCNU)** 100 mg/m² by slow I.V. infusion daily for 2 days; repeat dose q 6 weeks if platelet count above 100,000/mm³ and | *Cimetidine:* increased bone marrow suppression. Avoid use if possible. | Bone marrow suppression, including leukopenia and thrombocytopenia; nausea; vomiting; pain at infusion site; pulmonary fibrosis | Warn patient to watch for signs of infection and bone marrow suppression, such as fever, sore throat, anemia, fatigue, easy bruising, nose or gum bleeds, and tarry stools. Take temperature daily. To |

*(continued)*

## NEUROLOGIC DRUGS *(continued)*

| Drug, dosage, and route | Interactions | Adverse reactions | Special considerations |
|---|---|---|---|
| **Antineoplastics** *(continued)* | | | |
| **carmustine (BCNU)** *(continued)* white blood cell (WBC) count above 4,000/mm³ | | | reduce pain on infusion, dilute drug further or slow the infusion rate. If drug comes into contact with skin, wash off thoroughly (can cause brown stain). Solution is unstable in plastic I.V. bags; use only glass containers. |
| **lomustine (CCNU)** 130 mg/m² P.O. in a single dose q 6 weeks; give only if platelet count is above 100,000/mm³ and WBC count is above 4,000/mm³ | None significant. | Bone marrow suppression, including leukopenia and thrombocytopenia; nausea; vomiting | Give drug 2 to 4 hours after meals. To avoid nausea, give antiemetic before administering. Monitor blood counts weekly. Don't give more often than every 7 weeks; bone marrow suppression is cumulative and delayed. |
| **Antiparkinsonian drugs** | | | |
| **levodopa** 0.5 to 1 g P.O. daily b.i.d., t.i.d., or q.i.d. Increase dose by 0.75 g every 3 to 7 days; maximum dose—8 g daily | *Antacids:* may increase levodopa effect. *Anticholinergic drugs, tricyclic antidepressants, benzodiazepines, clonidine, papaverine, phenothiazines and other antipsychotics, phenytoin:* decreased levodopa effect. *Pyridoxine:* decreased levodopa effect. Check vitamin preparations and nutritional supplements for content of vitamin $B_6$ (pyridoxine). | Choreiform, dystonic and dyskinetic movements; involuntary grimacing; myoclonic body jerks; psychiatric disturbances; nausea; vomiting; anorexia; orthostatic hypotension | Adjust dose according to patient's response. Monitor vital signs, especially while adjusting dose. Warn patient and family not to increase drug dose without the doctor's orders. Warn patient of possible dizziness and orthostatic hypotension, especially at start of therapy. Inform patient and family that multivitamin preparations, fortified cereals, and certain over-the-counter drugs may contain pyridoxine (vitamin $B_6$), which can reverse the effects of levodopa. |
| **levodopa-carbidopa** 3 to 6 tablets of 25 mg carbidopa/250 mg levodopa P.O. daily in divided doses; maximum dose—8 tablets daily | *Papaverine, diazepam, clonidine, phenothiazines and other antipsychotics:* may antagonize antiparkinsonian actions. Use together cautiously. | Choreiform, dystonic, and dyskinetic movements; involuntary grimacing; myoclonic body jerks; orthostatic hypotension | Adjust dose according to patient's response. Drug effects occur more rapidly with levodopa-carbidopa than with levodopa alone. Monitor vital signs, especially while adjusting dose. If patient is receiving levodopa, discontinue this drug for at least 8 hours before starting levodopa-carbidopa. |

## NEUROLOGIC DRUGS *(continued)*

| Drug, dosage, and route | Interactions | Adverse reactions | Special considerations |
|---|---|---|---|
| *Antithrombotics* | | | |
| **aspirin** 1,300 mg P.O. daily | *Ammonium chloride (and other urine acidifiers):* increased aspirin levels. Monitor for aspirin toxicity. *Antacids in high doses (and other urine alkalinizers), corticosteroids:* decreased aspirin effect. *Oral anticoagulants and heparin:* increased risk of bleeding. | Prolonged bleeding time, nausea, vomiting, GI distress, and occult bleeding | Advise patients receiving large doses of aspirin for an extended period to watch for petechiae, bleeding gums, and GI bleeding, and to maintain adequate fluid intake. Give with food, milk, antacid, or water to reduce GI side effects. Obtain hemoglobin levels and prothrombin time periodically. |
| **dipyridamole** *For transient ischemic attacks:* 400 to 800 mg P.O. daily in divided doses | None significant. | Headache, dizziness, hypotension, nausea | Give 1 hour before meals. Monitor blood pressure and observe for side effects, especially with large doses. Also watch for signs of bleeding and for prolonged bleeding time. |
| **heparin** 7,500 to 10,000 units by I.V. bolus, then 1,000 units hourly by I.V. infusion | *Aspirin:* may increase bleeding risk. Don't use together. | Hemorrhage and excessive bleeding, thrombocytopenia | Measure partial thromboplastin time (PTT) carefully and regularly. Anticoagulation exists when PTT values are 1.5 to 2 times control values. When intermittent I.V. therapy is used, always draw blood 30 minutes before next scheduled dose to avoid spuriously elevated PTT. Avoid excessive I.M. injections of other drugs to prevent or minimize hematomas. |
| **sulfinpyrazone** *For transient ischemic attacks:* 600 to 800 mg P.O. daily in divided doses | *Oral anticoagulants:* possible bleeding. *Probenecid:* inhibited renal excretion of sulfinpyrazone. Use together cautiously. | Nausea, dyspepsia, epigastric pain | Give with milk, food, or antacid to reduce GI side effects. |
| **warfarin** maintenance dose—2 to 10 mg daily P.O. | *Allopurinol, chloramphenicol, danazol, clofibrate, diflunisal, dextrothyroxine, thyroid drugs, heparin, anabolic steroids, cimetidine, disulfiram, glucagon, in-* | Hemorrhage and excessive bleeding, dermatitis, skin rash, fever | Regularly measure PT to monitor anticoagulant effect. PT should be 1.5 to 2 times normal. When PT exceeds 2.5 times control value, bleeding risk is high. |

*(continued)*

## NEUROLOGIC DRUGS *(continued)*

| Drug, dosage, and route | Interactions | Adverse rections | Special considerations |
|---|---|---|---|
| **Antithrombotics** | | | |
| | *halation anesthetics, metronidazole, quinidine, influenza vaccine, sulindac, sulfonamides:* increased prothrombin time (PT). Monitor for bleeding. *Ethacrynic acid, indomethacin, mefenamic acid, oxyphenbutazone, phenylbutazone, salicylates:* increased PT; ulcerogenic effects. *Griseofulvin, haloperidol, carbamazepine, paraldehyde, rifampin:* reduced anticoagulant effect. *Glutethimide, chloral hydrate, sulfinpyrazone, triclofos sodium:* increased or decreased PT. | | Give drug at the same time daily. Stress importance of complying with recommended dose and keeping follow-up appointments. Advise patient to carry a card that identifies him as a potential bleeder. Also suggest that he use an electric razor when shaving to avoid scratching skin and to brush his teeth with a soft toothbrush. Female patients may report heavy menses. Fever and skin rash signal severe complications. Elderly patients and those with renal or hepatic failure are especially sensitive to warfarin effect. |
| **Heavy metal antagonists** | | | |
| **dimercaprol** 2 to 5 mg/kg by deep I.M. injection daily to q.i.d. | *131I uptake thyroid tests:* decreased iodine uptake. Don't schedule patient for this test during course of dimercaprol therapy. *Iron:* formed toxic metal complex. Don't use together. | Transient hypertension, tachycardia, nausea, vomiting, renal damage | Give only by deep I.M. route, and massage injection site after giving drug. Drug has an unpleasant, garlicky odor. Keep urine alkaline to prevent renal damage. Oral NaHCO₃ may be ordered. |
| **edetate calcium disodium** 1 g in 500 ml of 5% dextrose or 0.9% sodium chloride by I.V. infusion; 1 g I.M. | None significant. | Nephrotoxicity with acute tubular necrosis, fever, and chills 4 to 8 hours after infusion | Encourage fluids to promote excretion of edetate-metal complex (except in lead poisoning, since excess fluid may raise intracranial pressure). Monitor intake and output, urinalysis, blood urea nitrogen (BUN) level, and EKGs. To avoid toxicity, use drug with dimercaprol. Procaine HCl may be added to I.M. solutions to minimize pain. Avoid rapid I.V. infusions, and watch for local reactions afterward. |

## NEUROLOGIC DRUGS *(continued)*

| Drug, dosage, and route | Interactions | Adverse reactions | Special considerations |
|---|---|---|---|
| ***Miscellaneous*** | | | |
| **dexamethasone** *For cerebral edema:* 10 mg I.V., then 4 to 6 mg I.M. q 6 hours for 2 to 4 days; then decrease dose over 5 to 7 days | *Indomethacin, aspirin:* increased risk of GI distress and bleeding. Use together cautiously. | Atrophy at I.M. injection sites, euphoria, insomnia, peptic ulcer | Give I.M. injection deep into gluteal muscle. Avoid S.C. injections, which may result in atrophy and sterile abscesses. When possible, replace I.M. with P.O. route. |
| **disulfiram** *For chronic alcoholism:* 125 to 500 mg P.O. daily | *Alcohol:* disulfiram reaction (blurred vision, confusion, dyspnea, tachycardia, hypotension, flushing, nausea, vomiting, sweating, thirst, vertigo). *Isoniazid (INH):* ataxia or marked change in behavior. Avoid use. *Metronidazole:* psychotic reaction. Don't use together. *Paraldehyde:* toxic levels of acetaldehyde. Don't use together. | Drowsiness, headache, garlic-like taste, peripheral neuritis | Warn patient to avoid all alcohol, including that found in foods, medications like cough syrup and liniments, and toiletries like shaving lotion. Tell him that disulfiram reaction may occur as long as 2 weeks after single dose of disulfiram. The longer patient remains on drug, the more sensitive he becomes to alcohol. Blood alcohol level of 5 to 10 mg/dl may trigger a mild reaction; a level of 50 mg/dl a severe reaction; unconsciousness usually occurs at level of 125 to 150 ml/dl. Reaction may last ½ hour to several hours, or as long as alcohol remains in blood. Reassure patient that most side effects subside after 2 weeks of therapy. |
| **ergotamine** *For migraine headache:* 2 mg P.O. or S.L., then 1 to 2 mg P.O. hourly or S.L. q ½ hour. Maximum dose—6 mg daily | *Beta-adrenergic blockers:* possible increased vasoconstriction. | Numbness and tingling in fingers and toes, muscle pains | Most effective when used during prodromal stage of headache or as soon as possible after onset. Sublingual tablet is preferred during early stage of attack because of its rapid absorption. Prolonged exposure to cold weather should be avoided whenever possible. Cold may increase many of the side effects. Avoid prolonged administration and don't exceed recommended dosage. |

*(continued)*

## NEUROLOGIC DRUGS *(continued)*

| Drug, dosage, and route | Interactions | Adverse reactions | Special considerations |
|---|---|---|---|
| *Miscellaneous* | | | |
| **lactulose**<br>*For hepatic coma:*<br>20 to 30 g (30 to 45 ml) P.O. t.i.d. or q.i.d. until patient has two or three soft stools daily | None significant. | Cramps, belching, flatulence, diarrhea, hypernatremia | If desired, minimize drug's sweet taste by diluting with water or fruit juice or giving with food. Reduce dosage if diarrhea occurs. Replace fluid loss. Monitor serum sodium level for possible hypernatremia, especially with high doses. |
| **methysergide**<br>*For migraine headache prophylaxis:*<br>2 to 4 mg P.O. b.i.d. with meals | None significant. | Retroperitoneal and pulmonary fibrosis, vertigo, euphoria | Stop drug every 6 months; then restart after at least 3 or 4 weeks. Tell patient not to stop drug abruptly; may cause rebound headaches. Stop gradually over 2 to 3 weeks. Not for treatment of migraine or vascular headache in progress or for treatment of tension (muscle contraction) headaches. |
| **neomycin**<br>*For hepatic coma:*<br>1 to 3 g P.O. q.i.d. for 5 to 6 days | *Dimenhydrinate:* may mask symptoms of ototoxicity.<br>*Ethacrynic acid, furosemide:* increased ototoxicity.<br>*Other aminoglycosides, methoxyflurane:* increase ototoxicity and nephrotoxicity. | Ototoxicity, nephrotoxicity | Drug isn't absorbed at recommended dosage. However, more than 4 g of neomycin daily may be systemically absorbed and may lead to nephrotoxicity. Monitor renal function (urine output, specific gravity, BUN and creatinine levels, and creatinine clearance). Notify doctor of signs of decreasing renal function. |
| **propranolol**<br>*For migraine headache prophylaxis:*<br>160 to 240 mg P.O. daily in divided doses or once daily as sustained-release capsule | *Barbiturates, rifampin:* decreased effect of propranolol.<br>*Chlorpromazine, cimetidine:* increased effect of propranolol.<br>*Insulin, oral hypoglycemics:* monitor patient for altered dosage requirements. | Fatigue, lethargy, bradycardia, heart failure, heart block, hypotension | Monitor blood pressure for hypotension due to propranolol's beta-blocking action. To improve poor compliance with therapy, change dosage schedule to once or twice daily. Recognize that drug masks common signs of shock and hypoglycemia. Drug is for prophylaxis only; it won't effectively treat migraine already in progress. |

# Appendix: NANDA-Approved Nursing Diagnostic Categories

The following nursing diagnostic categories have been approved by the Seventh National Conference of the North American Nursing Diagnosis Association (NANDA)

Activity intolerance
Activity intolerance, Potential
Adjustment, Impaired
Airway clearance, Ineffective
Anxiety
Body temperature, Altered: Potential
Bowel elimination, Altered: Constipation
Bowel elimination, Altered: Diarrhea
Bowel elimination, Altered: Incontinence
Breathing Pattern, Ineffective
Cardiac output, Altered: Decreased
Comfort, Altered: Pain
Comfort, Altered: Chronic Pain
Communication, Impaired: Verbal
Coping, Family: Potential for growth
Coping, Ineffective family: Compromised
Coping, Ineffective family: Disabled
Coping, Ineffective individual
Diversional activity, Deficit
Family processes, Altered
Fear
Fluid volume deficit: Actual
Fluid volume deficit: Potential
Fluid volume excess
Gas exchange, impaired
Grieving, Anticipatory
Grieving, Dysfunctional
Growth and development, Altered
Health maintenance, Altered
Health maintenance management, Impaired
Hopelessness
Hyperthermia
Hypothermia
Incontinence, Functional
Incontinence, Reflex
Incontinence, Stress
Incontinence, Total
Incontinence, Urge
Infection: Potential for

Injury, Potential for
Injury, Potential for: Suffocating
Injury, Potential for: Poisoning
Injury, Potential for: Trauma
Knowledge deficit (specify)
Mobility, Impaired physical
Noncompliance (specify)
Nutrition, Altered: Less than body requirements
Nutrition, Altered: More than body requirements
Nutrition, Altered: Potential for more than body requirements
Parenting, Altered: Actual
Parenting, Altered: Potential
Post-trauma response
Powerlessness
Rape-trauma syndrome: Compound reaction
Rape-trauma syndrome: Silent reaction
Role performance, Altered
Self-care deficit: Bathing/hygiene
Self-care deficit: Dressing/grooming
Self-care deficit: Toileting
Self-care deficit: Feeding
Self-concept, Disturbance in: Body image
Self-concept, Disturbance in: Personal identity
Self-concept, Disturbance in: Self-esteem
Sensory/perceptual alterations: Visual, auditory, kinesthetic,
gustatory, tactile, olfactory
Sexual dysfunction
Sexuality, Altered patterns
Skin integrity, Impaired: Actual
Skin integrity, Impaired: Potential
Sleep pattern disturbance
Social interaction, Impaired
Social isolation
Spiritual distress (distress of the human spirit)
Swallowing, impaired
Thermoregulation, Ineffective
Thought processes, Altered
Tissue integrity, Impaired
Tissue integrity, Impaired: Oral mucous membrane
Tissue perfusion, Altered: Renal, cerebral, cardiopulmonary,
gastrointestinal, peripheral
Unilateral neglect
Urinary elimination, Altered patterns
Urinary retention
Violence, Potential for: Self-directed or directed at others

# Selected References

## Books
Braunwald, E., et al. *Harrison's Principles of Internal Medicine,* 11th ed. New York: McGraw-Hill Book Co., 1987.

Carpenito, L. *Nursing Diagnosis: Application to Clinical Practice.* Philadelphia: J.B. Lippincott Co., 1983.

Conway-Rutkowski, B. *Carini and Owens' Neurological and Neurosurgical Nursing,* 8th ed. St. Louis: C.V. Mosby Co., 1982.

Doenges, E., et al. *Nursing Care Plans: Nursing Diagnosis in Planning Patient Care.* Philadelphia: F.A. Davis Co., 1984.

Gilman, A., et al., eds. *Goodman and Gilman's The Pharmacological Basis of Therapeutics,* 6th ed. New York: Macmillan Publishing Co., 1980.

Nurse's Clinical Library. *Neurologic Disorders.* Springhouse, Pa.: Springhouse Corp., 1984.

Nurse's Reference Library. *Assessment.* Springhouse, Pa.: Springhouse Corp., 1983.

Snyder, M., ed. *A Guide to Neurological and Neurosurgical Nursing.* New York: John Wiley & Sons, 1983.

Snyder, M., and Jackle, M. *Neurologic Problems: A Critical Care Nursing Focus.* East Norwalk, Conn.: Appleton & Lange, 1980.

## Journals
Chase, M., and Whelan-Decker, E. "Nursing Management of a Patient with a Subarachnoid Hemorrhage," *Journal of Neurosurgical Nursing* 16(1):23-29, February 1984.

Ferido, T., and Habel, M. "Spasticity in Head Trauma and CVA Patients: Etiology and Management," *Journal of Neuroscience Nursing* 20(1):17-22, 1988.

Jackson, L. "Cerebral Vasospasm after an Intracranial Aneurysmal Subarachnoid Hemorrhage: A Nursing Perspective," *Heart & Lung* 15(1):14-22, January 1986.

Konikow, N. "Alterations in Movement: Nursing Assessment and Implications," *Journal of Neurosurgical Nursing* 17(1):61-65, February 1985.

McCash, A. "Meeting the Challenge of Craniotomy Care," *RN* 48(6):26-33, June 1985.

Mathewson, M. "Antidiuretic Hormone," *Critical Care Nurse* 6(5):88-93, September-October 1986.

Mathewson, M. "Ascending and Descending Spinal Cord Tracts," *Critical Care Nurse* 5(5):10-14, September-October 1985.

Metcalf, J. "Acute Phase Management of Persons with Spinal Cord Injury: A Nursing Diagnosis Perspective," *Nursing Clinics of North America* 21(4):589-98, December 1986.

Mitchell, P. "Intracranial Hypertension: Influence of Nursing Care Activities," *Nursing Clinics of North America* 21(4):563-76, December 1986.

Ozuna, J. "Alterations in Mentation: Nursing Assessment and Intervention," *Journal of Neurosurgical Nursing* 17(1):66-70, February 1985.

Walleck, C. "A Neurologic Assessment Procedure That Won't Make You Nervous," *Nursing82* 12(12):50-58, December 1982.

## Suggested Further Reading
Adams, R., and Victor, M. *Principles of Neurology,* 3rd ed. New York: McGraw-Hill Book Co., 1985.

Bubb, D. *Neurologic Problems.* Oradell, N.J.: Medical Economics Books, 1984.

Hanak, M., and Scott, A. *Spinal Cord Injury: An Illustrated Guide for Health Care Professionals.* New York: Springer Publishing Co., 1983.

Heimer, L. *The Human Brain and Spinal Cord.* New York: Springer-Verlag New York, 1983.

Hickey, J. *The Clinical Practice of Neurological and Neurosurgical Nursing,* 2nd ed. Philadelphia: J.B. Lippincott Co., 1985.

Kenner, C., et al. *Critical Care Nursing: Body, Mind, Spirit,* 2nd ed. Boston: Little, Brown & Co., 1985.

Kruse, M. *Nursing the Neurological and Neurotrauma Patient.* Totowa, N.J.: Rowman & Allanheld, 1986.

Liebman, M. *Neuroanatomy Made Easy and Understandable,* 3rd ed. Rockville, Md.: Aspen Publications, 1986.

Mitchell, P., et al. *Neurological Assessment and Nursing Practice.* East Norwalk, Conn.: Appleton & Lange, 1983.

"Nervous System," in *Patient Teaching,* Nurse's Reference Library. Springhouse, Pa.: Springhouse Corp., 1987.

Raimond, J., and Taylor, J. *Neurological Emergencies: Effective Nursing Care.* Rockville, Md.: Aspen Publications, 1985.

Rudy, E. *Advanced Neurological and Neurosurgical Nursing.* St. Louis: C.V. Mosby Co., 1984.

Scheinberg, P. *An Introduction to Diagnosis and Management of Common Neurologic Disorders,* 3rd ed. New York: Raven Press Pubs., 1986.

Zejdlik, C. *Management of Spinal Cord Injury.* Boston: Jones & Bartlett, 1983.

# Index

# Notes

# Notes

# Notes

# Notes

# Notes